BOSTON MEDICAL LIBRARY
in the Francis A. Countway
Library of Medicine ~ *Boston*

3282

ARISTOTLE'S WORKS.

THE WORKS OF ARISTOTLE,

THE FAMOUS PHILOSOPHER

CONTAINING,

HIS COMPLETE MASTERPIECE,

Displaying the Secrets of Nature in the Generation of Man:

TO WHICH IS ADDED,

THE FAMILY PHYSICIAN,

Being approved Remedies for the various Distempers incident to the Human Body:

ALSO

HIS EXPERIENCED MIDWIFE,

Absolutely necessary for Surgeons, Midwives, Nurses, and Childbearing Women:

AND

HIS LAST LEGACY,

Unfolding the Secrets of Nature in the Generation of Man.

A NEW AND IMPROVED EDITION,
With Engravings.

London:

PRINTED FOR MILLER, LAW, AND CARTER,
and sold by all the Booksellers.
1829.

INTRODUCTION.

If one of the meanest capacity were asked, What was the wonder of the world? I think the most proper answer would be, man; he being the little world, to whom all things are subordinate; agreeing in genius with sensitive things, all being animals, but different in the species: for man alone is endowed with reason; and therefore the Deity, at man's creation, (as the inspired penman tells us,) said, "Let us make man in our own image, after our own likeness." As if the LORD had said Let us make man in our image, that he, as a creature, may be like us: and the same in his likeness, that he may be after our image. Some of the fathers do distinguish, as if by the image the LORD doth plant the reasonable powers of the soul, will, and memory; and by likeness, the qualities of the mind, charity, justice, memory, &c. But Moses confounded this distinction, if you compare these texts of Scripture, Gen. i. 7, and v. 1, Colos. x. Eph. v. 14. And the apostle, where he saith, " He was created, after the image of God, in knowledge, and the same in righteousness."

The Greeks represent him as one turning his eyes upwards, towards him whose image and superscription he bears.

> See how the heavans' high Architect[d]
> Hath framed man in this wise,
> To stand, to go, to look erect,
> With body, face, and eyes?

And Cicero says, like Moses, all creatures were made to rot on the earth except man, to whom was given an upright frame to contemplate his Maker, and behold the mansion prepared for him above.

Now, to the end that so noble and glorious a creature might not quite perish, it pleased the Creator to give unto woman the field of generation, for the reception of human seed; whereby that natural and vegetable soul, which lies potentially in the seed, may by the plastic power, be reduced into act; that man, who is a mortal creature, by leaving his offspring behind him, may become immortal, and survive in his posterity. And because this field of generation, the womb, is the place where this excellent creature is formed, and in so wonderful a manner, that the royal Psalmist, having meditated thereon, cries out, as one in an ecstasy, "I am fearfully and wonderfully made!" it will be necessary to treat thereon in this book; which to that end is divided into two parts:

The first whereof treats of the manner and parts of generation in both sexes. For from the mutual desire they have to each other, which nature has implanted in them to that end, and from the delight which they take in the act of copulation, does the whole race of mankind proceed; and a particular account of what things are previous to that act; and also what are consequential to it; and how each member concerned is adapted and fitted for that work to which nature has designed it. And although, in uttering these things, something may be said which those that are unclean may make bad use of, and use it as a motive to stir up their bestial appetites; yet such may know that this never was intended for them; nor do I know any reason that those sober persons for whose use this was ment should want the help hereby designed them, because vain loose persons will be ready to abuse it.

The second part of this work is wholly designed for the female sex, and does treat largely not only of the distempers of the womb, and the various abuses, but also gives you proper remedies for the cure of them. For such is the ignorance of most women, that when by any distemper those parts are afflicted, they never know from whence it proceeds, nor how to apply a remedy: and such is their modesty also, that they are unwilling to ask that they may be informed. For the help of such is this designed: for, having my being from a woman, I thought none had more right to the grapes than she that planted the vine. And therefore, observing that, among all diseases incident to the body, there are none more frequent and perilous than those that do arise from the ill state of the womb; for through the evil quality thereof, the heart, the liver, and the brain are affected; from whence the actions, vital, natural, and animal, are hurt; and the virtues, concoctive, sanguificative, distributive, attractive, retentive, with the rest, are all weakened, so that from the womb come convulsions, epilepsies, apoplexies, palsies, and fevers, dropsies, malignant ulcers, &c. And there is no disease so bad, but may grow worse from the evil quality of it.

How necessary, therefore, is the knowledge of these things, let every unprejudiced reader judge: for, that many woman labour under them, through their ignorance and modesty (as I said before) woeful experience makes manifest. Here, therefore, as in a mirror, they may be made acquainted with their own distempers, and have suitable remedies without applying themselves to physicians, to which they have so great reluctance.

ARISTOTLE'S MASTER-PIECE

PART FIRST.

CHAPTER I.

Of Marriage, and at what Age Young Men and Virgins are capable of it; and why so much desire it. Also, how long Men and Women are capable of having Children.

THERE are very few, except some Profest debauchees, but what will readily agree, that " Marriage is honourable to all," being ordained by Heaven in paradise; and without which no man or woman can be in a capacity, honestly, to yield obedience to the first law of the creation, " Increase and multiply." And since it is natural in young people to desire these mutual embraces, proper to the marriage bed, it behoves parents to look after their children, and, when they find them inclinable to marriage, not violently to restrain their affections, and oppose their inclinations (which, instead of allaying them, makes them but the more impetuous,) but rather provide such suitable matches for them, as may make their lives comfortable : lest the crossing of their inclinations should precipitate them to commit those follies that may bring an indelible stain upon their families.

The inclinations of maids to marriage is to be known by many symptoms; for, when they arrive at puberty, which is about the 14th or 15th year of their age, then their natural purgations begin to flow: and the blood, which is no longer taken to augment their bodies, abounding, stirs up their minds to venery. External causes also may incite them to it: for their spirits being brisk and inflamed, when they arrive at that age, if they eat hard salt things and spices, the body becomes more and more heated, whereby the desire to venereal embraces is very great and sometimes almost insuperable. And the use of this so much desired enjoyment being denied to Virgins, many times is followed by dismal consequences; such as the green wesel colonet, short breathing, trembling of the heart, &c. But when they are married, and their venereal desires satisfied by the enjoyment of their husbands, those distempers vanish, and they become more gay and lively than before. Also, their eager staring at men, and effecting their company, shews that nature pushes them upon coition; and their parents neglecting to provide them with husbands, they break through modesty to satisfy themselves in unlawful embraces. It is the same with brisk widows: who cannot be satisfied without that benevolence to which they were accustomed when they had husbands.

At the age of 14, the menses, in virgins, begin to flow, when they are capable of conceiving, and continue, generally, to 44, when they cease bearing, unless their bodies are strong and healthful, which sometime enables them to bea at 55. But many times the menses proceed from some violence done to nature, or some morbific matter, which often proves fatal. And, therefore, men who are desirous of issue ought to marry a woman within the age aforesaid, or blame themselves if they meet with disappointment: if an old man not worn out by diseases and incontinency, marry a brisk lively lass, there is hope of his having children to seventy or eighty years.

Hipprocrates says, that a youth of 15, or between that and 17, having much vital strength, is capable of getting children; and also, that the force of procreating matter increases till 45, 50, and 55, and then begins to flag; the seed, by degrees, becoming unfruitful, the natural spirits being extinguished and the humours dried up. Thus in general, but as to particulars it often falls out otherwise. Nay, it is reported by a reditable author that in Sweden, a man was married at 100 years of age to a girl of 30 years, and had many children by her; but his countenance was so fresh, that those who knew him not, imagined him not to exceed 50. And in Campania where the air is clear and temperate, men of 80 marry young virgins, and have children by them; which shows, that age in them hinders not procreation, unless they be exhausted in their youth and their yards shrivelled up.

If any would know why a woman is sooner barren than a man, they may be assured that the natural heat, which is the cause of generation, is more predominant in the latter than in the former; for since a woman is truly more moist than a man as her monthly purgations demonstrate, as also the softness of her body; it is also apparent, that he doth much exceed her in natural heat, which is the chief thing that concocts the humours into proper aliment, which the woman wanting grows fat: when a man, through his native heat, melts his fat by degrees, and his humours are dissolved; and, by the benefit thereof, are elaborated into seed. And this may also be added, that women, generally, are not so strong as men, nor so wise or prudent; nor have so much reason and ingenuity in ordering affairs; which shows, that thereby their faculties are hindered in operation.

CHAPTER II.

How to get a Male or Female Child; and of the Embryo and perfect Birth; and the fittest Time for Copulation.

WHEN a young couple is married, they naturally desire children, and therefore use the means that nature has appointed to that end. But notwithstanding their endeavours, they must know. the success of all depends on the blessing of GOD: not only so, but the sex, whether male or female, is from his disposal also: though it cannot be denied, but secondary causes have influence therein, especially two First, the genital humour, which is brought by the arteria præparantes to the testes, in form of blood, and there elaborated into seed, by the seminifical faculty residing in them. Secondly, the desire of coition, which fires the imagination with unusual fancies, and by the sight of brisk charming beauty may soon inflame the appetite. But if nature be enfeebled, such meats must be eaten as will conduce to afford such aliment as makes the seed abound, and restores the decays of nature, that the faculties may freely operate, and remove impediments obstructing the procreation of children.

Then, since diet alters the evil state of the body to a better, those subject to barrenness must eat such meats as are juicy and nourish well, making the body lively and full of sap: of which faculty are all hot moist meats. For, according to Galen, seed is made of pure concocted and windy superfluity of blood; whence we may conclude, there is a power in many things to accumulate seed, and also to augment it, and other things of force to cause erection, as hen eggs, pheasants, woodcocks, gnat snappers, thrushes, blackbirds, young pigeons, sparrows, partridges, capons, almonds, pine nuts, raisins, currants, strong wines taken sparingly, especially those made of the grapes of Italy. But erection is chiefly caused by scuraum, eringoes, cresses, crysmon, parsnips, artichokes, turnips, asparagus, candied ginger, galings, acorns bruised to powder and drank in muscadel, scallion, and sea shell fish, &c. But these must have time to perform their operation, and must use them for a considerable time, or you will reap but little benefit by them. The act of coition being over, let the woman repose herself on her right side, with her head lying low, and her body declining, that by sleeping in that posture, the cani, on the right side of the matrix, may prove the place of the conception: for therein is the greatest generative heat, which is the chief procuring cause of male children, and rarely fails the expectation of those that experience it, especially if they do but keep warm, without much motion, leaning to the right, and drinking a little spirit of saffron and juice of hyssop in a glass of malaga or alicant, when they lie down and arise for a week.

For a female child, let the woman lie on her left side, strongly fancying a female in the time of procreation, drinking the decoction of female mercury four days, from the first day of purgation; the male mercury having the like operation in case of a male: for this concoction purges the right and left side of the womb, opens the receptacles, and makes way for the seminary of generation. The best time to beget a female is, when the moon is in the wane, in Libra, or Aquarius. Advicene says, when the menses are spent and the womb cleansed, which is commonly in five or seven days at most, if a man lie with his wife from the first day she is purged to the fifth, she will conceive a male; but from the fifth to the eighth a female; and from the eighth to the twelfth, a male again; but after that, perhaps neither distinctly, but both in an hermaphrodite. In a word, they that would be happy in the fruits of their labour, must observe to use copulation in due distance of time, not too often nor too seldom, for both are alike hurtful; and to use it immoderately weakens and wastes the spirits, and spoils the seed. And thus much for

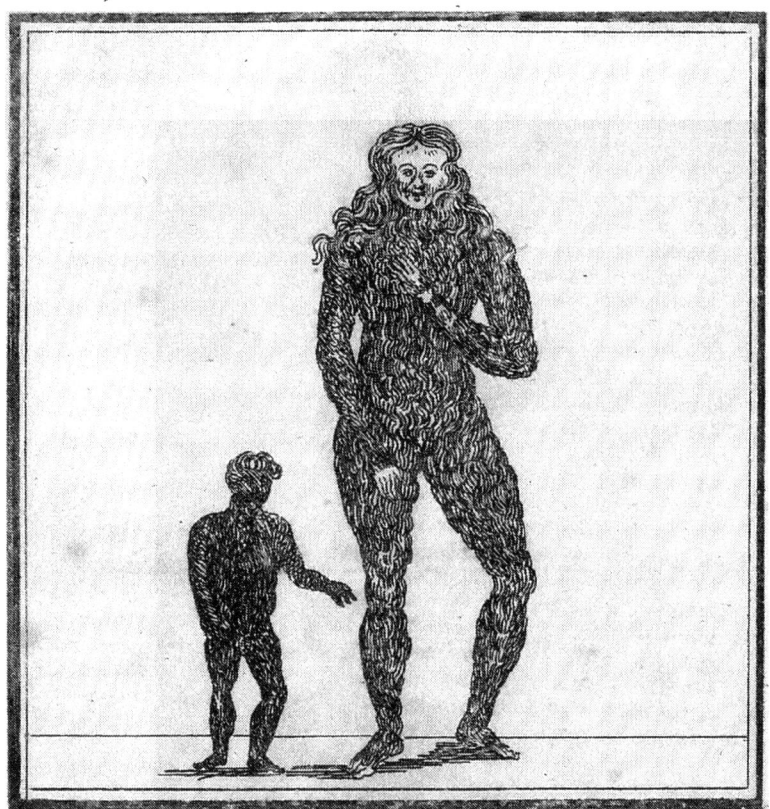

Page 17.

EFFIGIES OF A MAID AND INFANT, That were born black and covered with Hair by the Imagination of the Parents.

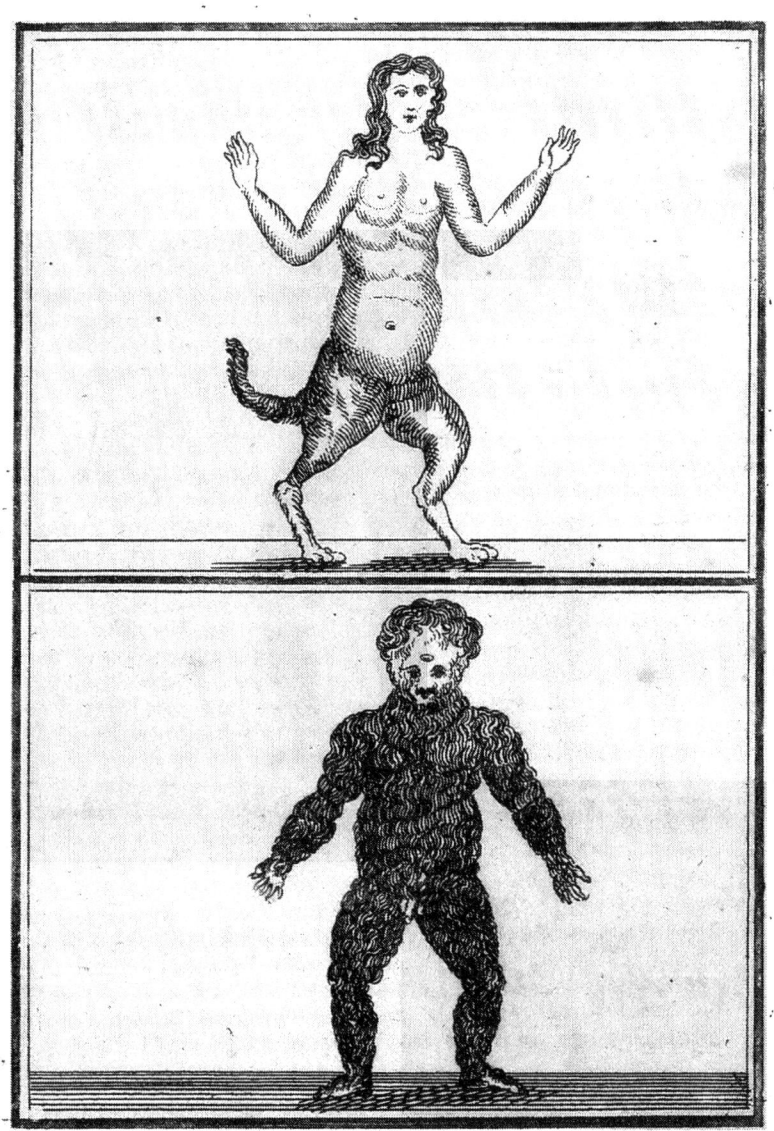

Where children thus are born with hary coats
Heaven's wrath unto the kingdom it denotes.

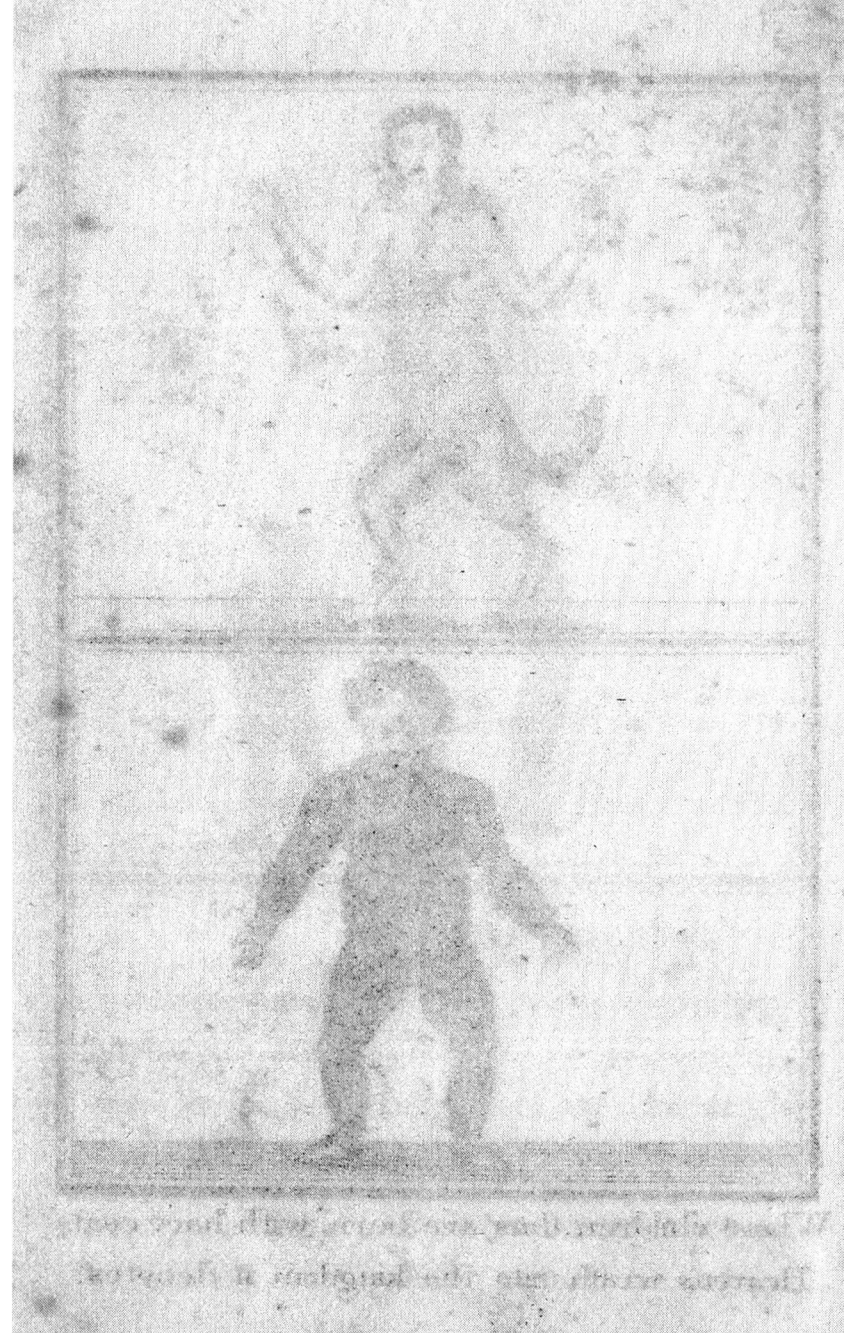

Two children, hand in hand, with faces east.
Dances with me. The Kingdom is light of.

the first particular. The second is, to let the reader know how the child is formed in the womb, what accident it is liable to there, and how nourished and brought forth. There are various opinions concerning this matter, therefore I shall show what the learned say about it.

Man consists of an egg, which is impregnated in the testicles of the woman, by the more subtle part of the man's seed; but the forming faculty and virtue in the seed is a divine gift, it being abundantly endued with a vital spirit, which gives sap and form to the embryo: so that all parts and bulk of the body, which is made up in a few months, and gradually formed into the lovely figure of a man, do consist in, and are adumbrated thereby, most sublimely expressed, Psalm cxxxix, "I will praise thee, O Lord, for I am fearfully and wonderfully made."

Physicians have remarked four different times, in which a man is framed and perfected in the womb: the first moon after coition, being perfected in the first week, if no flux happens; which sometimes falls out through the slipperness of the head of the matrix, that shifts over like a rose-bud, and opens suddenly. The second time of forming is assigned, when nature makes manifest mutation in the conception, so that all the substance seems congealed flesh and blood, and happens 12 or 14 days after copulation. And though this fleshy mass abounds with inflamed blood, yet remains undistinguishable, without form, and may be called an embryo, and compared to seed sown in the ground, which, through heat and moisture, grows by degrees, to a perfect form, in plant or grain. The third time assigned to make up this fabric is, when the principal parts show themselves plain: as the heart, whence proceed the arteries: the brain, from which the nerves, like small threads run through the whole body; and the liver, that divides the chyle from the blood, brought to it by the venna porta. The two first are fountains of life, that nourish every part of the body: in framing which, the faculty of the womb is busied, from the conception to the eighth day of the first month. The fourth and last, about the thirtieth day, the outward parts are seen nicely wrought, distinguished by joints. From which time, it is no longer an embryo, but a perfect child.

Most males are perfect by the thirtieth day, but females seldom to the forty-second or forty-fifth day; because the heat of the womb is greater in producing the male than the female. And, for the same reason, a woman going with a male child, quickens in three months: but going with a female, rarely under four: at which time its hair and nails come forth; and the child begins to stir, kick, and move in the womb; and then the woman is troubled with a loathing of her meat; and greedy longing for things contrary to nutriment, as coals, rubbish, chalk &c. which desire often occasions abortion and miscarriage. Some women have been so extravagant as to long for hob nails, leather, man's flesh, horse flesh, and other unnatural as well as unwholesome food: for want of which thing, they have either miscarried, or the child has continued dead in the womb for many days, to the imminent hazard of their lives. But I shall now proceed to show by what real means the child is sustained in the womb, and what posture it there remains in.

Various are the opinions about nourishing the fœtus in the womb. Some say by blood only, from the umbilical vein; others, by chyle taken in by the mouth. But it is nourished diversely, according to the several degrees of perfection: and an egg passes from a conception to a fœtus ready for birth. But, first, let us explain the meaning of the ovum or egg. In the generation of the fœtus, there are two principles, active and passive; the active is the man's seed, elaborated in the testicles, out of the arterial blood and animal spirits; the passive is an egg, impregnated by the man's seed. The nature of conception is thus: the most spirituous part of man's seed, in the act of generation, reaching up to the testicles of the woman, which contain divers eggs, impregnates one of them; and being conveyed by the ovaducts to the bottom of the womb presently begins to swell bigger and bigger, and drinks in the moisture that is plentifully sent thither, as seeds suck moisture in the ground to make them sprout out. When the parts of the embryo begin to be a little more perfect, and that, at the same time, the chorin is so very thick, that the liquor cannot soak through it, the umbilical vessels begin to be formed, and to extend the side of the amnion, which they pass through, and all through the aliantreides and chorin, and are implanted in the placenta: which gathering upon the chorin, joins to the uterus. And now the arteries that before sent out the nourishment into the cavity of the womb, open by the orifice into the placenta, where they deposit the said juice, which is drunk up by the umbilical vein: conveyed by it to the liver of the fœtus, then to the heart, where its thin and spirituous part is turned into blood, while the groosser part, descending by the aorta, enters the umbilical arteries, and is discharged into its cavity by those branches that run through the amnion.

As soon as the mouth, stomach, gullet, &c. are formed so perfectly, that the fœtus can swallow, it sucks in some of the grosser nutricious juice that is deposited in the amnion by the umbilical arteries, which, descending into the stomach and intestines, is received by the lacteal veins, as in adult persons.

The fœtus being perfected, at the time before specified, in all parts, it lies equally balanced in the centre of the womb, on its head; and being long turned over, so that the head a little inclines, it lays its chin upon its breast, its heels and ankles upon its buttocks, its hands on its cheeks, and its thumbs to its eyes: but its legs and thighs are carried upwards, with its hams bending, so that they touch the bottom of its belly; the former, and that part of the body which is over against us, as the forehead, nose and face, are towards the mother's back, the head inclining downwards towards the rump-bone that joins to the os sacrum; which bone, together with the os pubis, in the time of birth, is loosed

The learned Hippocrates affirms, that the child as he is placed in the womb, hath his hands on his knees and his head bent to his feet; so that he lies round together, his hands upon his knees, and his face between them; so that each eye touches each thumb, and his nose betwixt his knees. And of the same opinion, in this matter, war Bartholinus Columbus is of opinion, that the figure of the child in the womb is round, the right arm bowed, the fingers under the ear and above the neck, the head bowed, so that the chin toucheth the breast, the left arm bowed above both breast and face, and propped up by the bending of the right elbow; the legs are lifted upwards, the right so much that the thigh toucheth the belly, the knees the navel, the heel toucheth the left buttock, and the foot is turned back, and covereth the secrets: the left thigh toucheth the belly, and the leg lifted up to the breast; as below.

CHAPTER III.

The Reason why Children are like their Parents, and that the Mother's Imagination contributes thereto: and whether the Man or Woman is the cause of the Male or Female Child.

In the case of similitude, nothing is more powerful than the imagination of the mother: for if she fix her eyes upon any object, it will so impress her mind, that it ofttimes so happens that the child has a representation thereof on some part of its body. And if, in the act of copulation, the woman earnestly look upon the man, and fix her mind upon him, the child will resemble its father. Nay, if a woman, even in unlawful copulation, fix her mind on her husband, the child will resemble him, though he did not beget it. The same effect hath imagination in occasioning warts, stains, mole spots and dartes; though indeed they sometimes happen through frights, or extravagant longing. Many women, being with child, on seeing a hare cross the road before them, will, through the force of imagination, bring forth a child with a hairy lip. Some children are born with flat noses and wry mouths, great blubber lips, and ill shaped bodies: which must be ascribed to the imagination of the mother, who hath cast her eyes and mind upon some ill shaped creature.— Therefore it behoves all women with child, if possible, to avoid such sights, or, at least, not to regard them. But though the mother's imagination may contribute much to the features of the child, yet, in manners, wit, and propension of the mind, experience tells us, that children are commonly of the condition with their parents and same tempers. But the vigour or disability of persons in the act of copulation many times causes it to be otherwise: for children got through the heat and strength of desire, must needs partake more of the nature and inclinations of their parents, than those begotten with desires more weak: and therefore, the children, begotten by men in their old age, are generally weaker than those begotten by them in their youth. As to the share which each of the parents has in begetting the child, we will give the opinion of the ancients about it.

Though it is apparent, say they, that the man's seed is the

chief efficient beginning of the action, motion, and generation; yet that the woman affords seed, and effectually contributes in that point to the procreation of the child, is evinced by strong reasons. In the first place, seminary vessels had been given her in vain, and genical testicles inverted, if the woman wanted seminal excrescence, for nature does nothing in vain and therefore we must grant they are made for the use of seed and procreation and placed in their proper parts, both the testicles and receptacles of seed, whose nature is to operate and afford virtue to the seed. And to prove this, there needs no stronger argument, say they, than that if a woman do not use copulation to eject her seed, she often falls into strange diseases as appears by young women and virgins. A second reason they urge is, that although the society of a lawful bed consists not altogether in these things, yet it is apparent the female sex are never better pleased, nor appear more blythe and jocund, than when they are satisfied this way: which is an inducement to believe, they have more pleasure and titulation therein than men. For, since nature causes much delight to accompany ejection, by the breaking forth of the swelling spirits, and the swiftness of the nerves; in which case, the operation on the woman's part is double, she having an enjoyment both by ejection and reception, by which she is more delighted in the act.

Hence it is, say they, that the child more frequently resembles the mother than the father, because the mother contributes most towards it. And they think it may be further instanced, from the endeared affection they bear them: for that besides their contributing seminal matter, they feed and nourish the child with the purest fountain of blood, until its birth. Which opinion Galen affirms, by allowing children to participate most of the mother; and ascribes the difference of sex to the operation of the menstrual blood; but the reason of the likeness, he refers to the power of the seed: for, as the plants receive more nourishment from fruitful ground, than from the industry of the husbandman; so the infant receives more abundance from the mother than the father. For the seed of both is cherished in the womb, and there grows to perfection, being nourished with blood. And for this reason it is, say they, that children, for the most part, love their mother best, because they receive the most of their substance from their mother: for about nine months she nourishes her child in the womb with her purest blood; then her love towards it newly born, and its likeness, do clearly show, that the woman affordeth seed, and contributes more towards making the child than the man.

But in all this the ancients were very erroneous; for the

testicles, so called in women, afford not any seed, but are two eggs, like those of fowls, and other creatures: neither have they any office, as those of men, but are indeed the ovaria, wherein the eggs are nourished by the sanguinary vessels dispersed through them; and from thence one or more, as they are fecundated by the man's seed, is separated and conveyed into the womb by the ovaducts. The truth of this is plain, for if you boil them, their liquor will be the same colour, taste, and consistency with the taste of bird eggs. If any object that they have no shells, that signifies nothing: for the eggs of fowls, while they are in the ovary, nay, after they had fastened into the uterus, have no shell. And though, when they are laid, they have one, yet that is no more than a defence which nature has provided them against any outward injury, while they are hatched without the body: whereas those of women being hatched within the body, need no other fence than the womb, by which they are sufficiently secured. And this is enough, I hope, for the clearing of this point.

As for the third thing proposed, as whence grow the kind, and whether the man or woman is the cause of the male or female infant.—The primary cause we must ascribe to GOD, as is most justly his due, who is the Ruler and Disposer of all things; yet he suffers many things to proceed according to the rules of nature, by their inbred motion, according to usual and natural courses, without variation: though indeed by favour from on high. Sarah conceived Isaac; Hannah, Samuel: and Elizabeth, John the Baptist: but these were all very extraordinary things, brought to pass by a divine power above the course of nature: nor have such instances been wanting in latter days; therefore I shall wave them, and proceed to speak of things natural.

The ancient physicians and philosophers say, that since there are two principles out of which the body of man is made, and which render the child like the parents, and by one or other of the sex, viz. seed common to both sexes, and menstrual blood, proper to the woman only: the similitude, say they, must needs consist in the force and virtue of the male or female: so that it proves like the one or other, according to the quantity afforded by either; but that the difference of the sex is not referred to the seed, but to the menstrual blood, which is proper to the woman, is apparent; for, were that force altogether retained in the seed, the male seed being of the hottest quality, male children would abound, and few of the female be propagated: wherefore the sex is attributed to the temperament of the active qualities, which consist in heat and cold, and the nature of the matter under them—that is, the flowing of the menstruous blood; but now the seed, say they, affords both force to procreate and form the child, and matter for its generation; and in the menstruous blood there is both matter and force; for as the seed most helps the material principle, so also does the menstrual blood the potential seed: which is, says Galen, blood well concocted by the vessels that contain it. So that blood is not only the matter of generating the child, but also seed, it being impossible that menstrual blood hath both principles.

The ancients also say, that the seed is the stronger efficient, the matter of it being very little in quantity, but the potential quality of it is very strong, wherefore, if these principles of generation, according to which the sex is made, were only, say they, in the menstrual blood, then would the children be all mostly females: as, were the efficient force in the seed, they would be all males; but since both have operation in menstrual blood, matter predominates in quantity, and in the seed force and virtue. And therefore Galen thinks the child receives its sex rather from the mother than from the father; for though his seed contributes a little to the material principle, yet it is more weakly. But for likeness, it is referred rather to the father than to the mother. Yet the woman's seed receiving strength from the menstrual blood for the space of nine months, overpowers the man's as to that particular, for the menstrual blood flowing in vessels, rather cherishes the one than the other: from which it is plain, the woman affords both matter to make, and force and virtue to perfect the conception: though the female's seed be fit nutriment for the male's, by reason of the thinness of it, being more adapted to make up conception thereby. For as of soft wax and moist clay the artificer can frame what he intends, so say they, the man's seed mixing with the woman's, and also with the menstrual blood, helps to make the form and perfect part of man.

But, with all imaginable deference to the wisdom of our fathers, give me leave to say, that their ignorance in the anatomy of man's body hath led them into the paths of error, and run them into great mistakes. For their hypothesis of the formation of the embryo, from cotomixture of seed, and the nourishment of it too in the menstruous blood, being wholly false, their opinion, in this case, must of necessity be so likewise.

I shall therefore conclude this chapter with observing, that although a strong imagination of the mother may often determine the sex, yet the main agent in this case is the plastic or formative principle, according to those laws and rules given to us by the wise Creator, who makes and fashions it, and therein determines the sex, according to the council of his will.

CHAPTER IV.

That Man's Soul is not propagated by the Parents, but is infused by its Creator and can neither die nor corrupt. At what time it is infused. Of its Immortality, and Certainty of its Resurrection.

MAN's soul is of so divine a nature and excellency, that man himself cannot comprehend it, being the infused breath of the Almighty, of an immortal nature, and not to be comprehended but by him that gave it. For Moses by holy inspiration, relating the original of man, tells us, that "God breathed into his nostrils the breath of life, and he became a living soul." Now, as for all other creatures, at his word they were made, and had life: but the creature that God had set over his works was his peculiar workmanship; formed by him out of the dust of the earth and he condescended to breathe into his nostrils the breath of life; which seems to denote both care, and, if we may so term it, labour, used about man more than about all other creatures; he only partaking and participating of the blessed divine nature, bearing God's image in innocence and purity, whilst he stood firm: and when, by his fall, that lively image was defaced, yet such was the love of the Creator towards him, that he found out a way to restore him: the only begotten Son of the eternal Father coming into the world to destroy the works of the devil, and to raise up man from that low condition to which his sin and fall had reduced him, to a state above that of angels.

If, therefore, man would understand the excellency of his soul, let him turn his eyes inwardly, and look into himself, and search diligently his own mind: and there he shall see many admirable gifts and excellent ornaments, that must needs fill him with wonder and amazement: as reason, understanding, freedom of will, memory, &c. that plainly show the soul to be descended from a heavenly original: and that therefore it is of an infinite duration, and not subject to annihilation Yet, for its many offices and operations whilst in the body, it goes under several denominations: for, when it enlivens the body, it is called the soul; when it gives knowledge, the judgment of the mind; and when it recalls things past, the memory; whilst it discourses and discerns, reason; whilst it contemplates, the spirit; while it is in the sensitive parts, the senses. And these are the principal offices, whereby the soul declares its powers, and performs its action. For being seated in the highest parts of the body, it diffuseth its force into every member. It is not propagated from the parents, nor mixed with gross matter, but the infused breath of GOD, immediately proceeding from him: not passing from one to another as was the opinion of Pythagoras, who held a transmigration of the soul: but that the soul is given to every infant by infusion, is the most received and orthodox opinion. And the learned do likewise agree, that this is done when the infant is perfected in the womb, which happens about the 24th day after conception: especially for males, who are generally born at the end of nine months: but in females, who are not so soon formed and perfected through defect of heat, not till the 50th day. And though this day, in all cases, cannot be truly set down, yet Hippocrates has given his opinion, that it is so when the child is formed, and begins to move, when born in due season. In his book of the nature of infants, he says, if it be a male, and he be perfect on the the 30th day, and move on the 70th, he will be born on the 7th month: but if he be perfectly formed on the 35th day, he will move on the 70th, and be born in the 8th month. Again, if he be perfectly formed on the 45th day, he will move on the 90th, and be born in the 9th month. Now, from these passing of days and months, it plainly appears, that tne day of forming being doubled, makes up the day of moving, and that day, three times reckoned, makes up the day of birth. As thus, when 35 perfects the form, if you double it, makes 70 the day of motion: and 3 times 70 amounts to 210 days; which, allowing 30 days to a month, make 7 months; and so you must consider the rest. But as to a female, the case is different: for it is longer perfecting in the womb, the mother ever going longer with a girl than a boy, which makes the account differ, for a female formed in 30 days, moves not till the 70th day, and is born in the 7th month: when she is formed on the 40th, she moves not till the 80th, and is born in the 8th month: but if she be perfectly formed on the 45th day, she moves on the 90th, and is born in the 9th month; but if she that is formed on the 60th day, moves the 110th day, she will be born in the 10th month. I treat the more largely hereof, that the reader may know that the reasonable soul is not propagated by the parents, but is infused by the Almighty, when the child hath its perfect form, and is exactly distinguished in its lineaments.

Now, as the life of every other creature, as Moses shows, is in the blood, so the life of man consisteth in the soul, which, although subject to passion by reason of the gross composures of the body, in which it has a temporary confinement, yet it is immortal, and cannot in itself corrupt or suffer change, it being a spark of the Divine Mind. And that every man has a peculiar soul plainly appears by the vast difference between the will, judgment, opinion, manners, and affections in men. This David observes, when he says, "GOD hath fashioned the hearts and minds of men; and has given to every one his own being, and a soul of its own nature." Hence Solomon rejoiced that GOD had given him a soul, and a body agreeable to it. It has been disputed among the learned, in what part of the body the soul resides: some are of opinion, its residence is in the middle of the heart, and from thence communicates itself to every part; which Solomon (Prov. iv.) seems to confirm, when he says, "Keep thy heart with all diligence, for out of it are the issues of live." But many curious physicians, searching the works of nature in man's anatomy, do affirm that its chief seat is in the brain, from whence proceed the senses, faculties, and actions, diffusing the operation of the soul through all the parts of the body whereby it is enlivened with heat and force to the heat, by the arteries, corodities, or sleepy arteries, which part upon the throat: the which, if they happen to be broke or cut, they cause barrenness, and if stopped an apoplexy: for their must necessarily be ways through which the spirits, animal and vital, may have intercourse and convey native heat from the soul. For, though the soul has its chief seat in one place, it operates in every part, exercising every member, which are the soul's instruments by which she discovers her power, But if it happen that any of the organical parts are out of tune, its whole work is confused, as appears in idiots and madmen; though in some of them the soul, by a vigorous exertion of its power, recovers its innate strength, and they become right after a long despondency in mind: but in others it is not recovered again in this life. For, as fire under ashes, or the sun obscured from our sight by thick clouds, afford not their lawful lustre, so the soul, overwhelmed in moist or morbid matter, is darkened, and reason thereby over clouded: and though reason shines less in children than in such as are arrived to maturity, yet no man must imagine that the soul of an infant grows up with the child, for then would it again decay; but it suits itself to nature's weakness, and the imbecility of the body wherein it is placed, that it may operate the better. And as the body is more and more capable of receiving its influence, so the soul does more and more exert its faculties, having force and endowments at the time it enters the form of a child in the womb; for its substance can receive nothing less. And thus much to prove that the soul comes not from the parents, but is infused by GOD. I shall next prove its immortality, and so domonstrate the certainty of our resurrection.

Of the Immortality of the Soul.

THAT the soul of man is a divine ray, infused by the Sovereign Creator, I have already proved, and now come to show, that whatever immediately proceeds from him, and participates of his nature, must be as immortal as its original; for though all other creatures are endowed with life and motion, yet they want a reasonable soul; and from thence it is concluded that their life is in their blood, and that being coruptible, they perish and are no more: but man being endowed with a reasonable soul, and stamped with the Divine image its of a different nature; and though his body be corruptible, yet his soul being of an immortal nature, cannot perish; but must, at the dissolution of his body, return to God, who gave it either to receive reward or punishment. Now, that the body can sin of itself is impossible, because, wanting the soul, which is the principle of life, it cannot act nor proceed to any thing either good or evil: for could it do so, it might even sin in the grave: but it is plain, that after death there is a cessation. for as death leaves us, so judgment will find us.

Now, reason having evidently demonstrated the soul's immortality, the Holy Scriptures do abundantly give testimony of the truth of the resurrection: as the reader may see by perusing the 14th and 19th chapters of Job, and 5th of John. I shall therefore leave the further discoursing of this matter to divines, whose proper province it is, and return to treat of the works of nature.

CHAPTER V.

Of Monsters and monstrous Births; and the several reasons thereof, according to the opinion of the Ancients. Also, whether Monsters are endowed with reasonable Souls; and whether Devils can engender; is here briefly discussed.

By the Ancients, monsters are ascribed to depraved conceptions, and are designated to be excursions of nature, which are vicious one of these four ways: either in figure, magnitude, situation, or number.

In figure, when a man bears the character of a beast, as did the beast in Saxony. In magnitude, when one part doth not equalize with another; as when one part is too big or too little for the other parts of the body. But this is so common among us, that I need not produce a testimony for it.

I proceed to explain the cause of their generation, which is either divine or natural. The divine cause proceeds from God's permissive will, suffering parents to bring forth abominations for their filthy and corrupt affections, which are let loose unto wickedness, like brute beast that have no understanding. Wherefore it was enacted among the ancient Romans, that those who were in any way deformed, should not be admitted into religious houses. And St. Jerome was grieved, in his time, to see the deformed and lame offering up spiritual sacrifices to God in religious houses. And Keckerman, by way of inference, excludeth all that are ill shaped from this presbyterian function in the church. And that which is of more force than all, God himself commanded Moses not to receive such to offer sacrifice among his people; and he renders the reason, Lev. xxii, 28. "Lest he pollute my sanctuaries." Because the outward deformity of the body is often a sign of the pollutions of the heart, as a curse laid upon the child for the incontinence of the parents. Yet it is not always so. Let us therefore duly examine, and search out the natural cause of their generation: which (according to the ancients, who have dived into the secrets of nature,) is either in the matter or in the agent; in the seed, or in the womb.

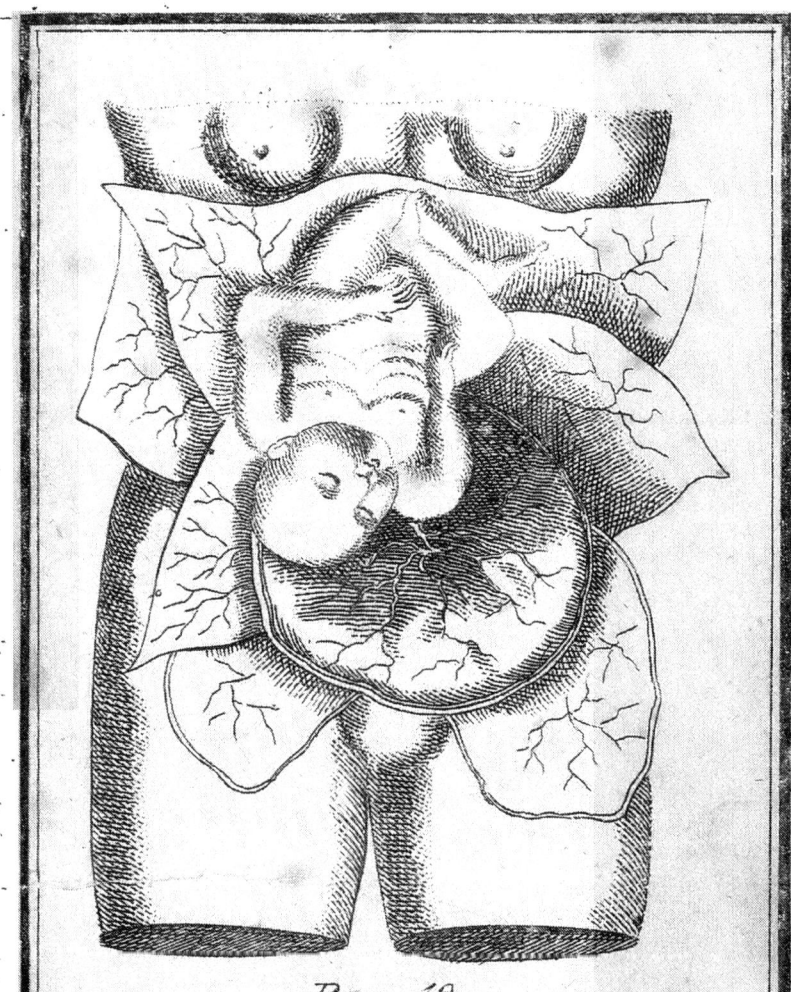

Page 19.
FORM OF A CHILD IN THE WOMB

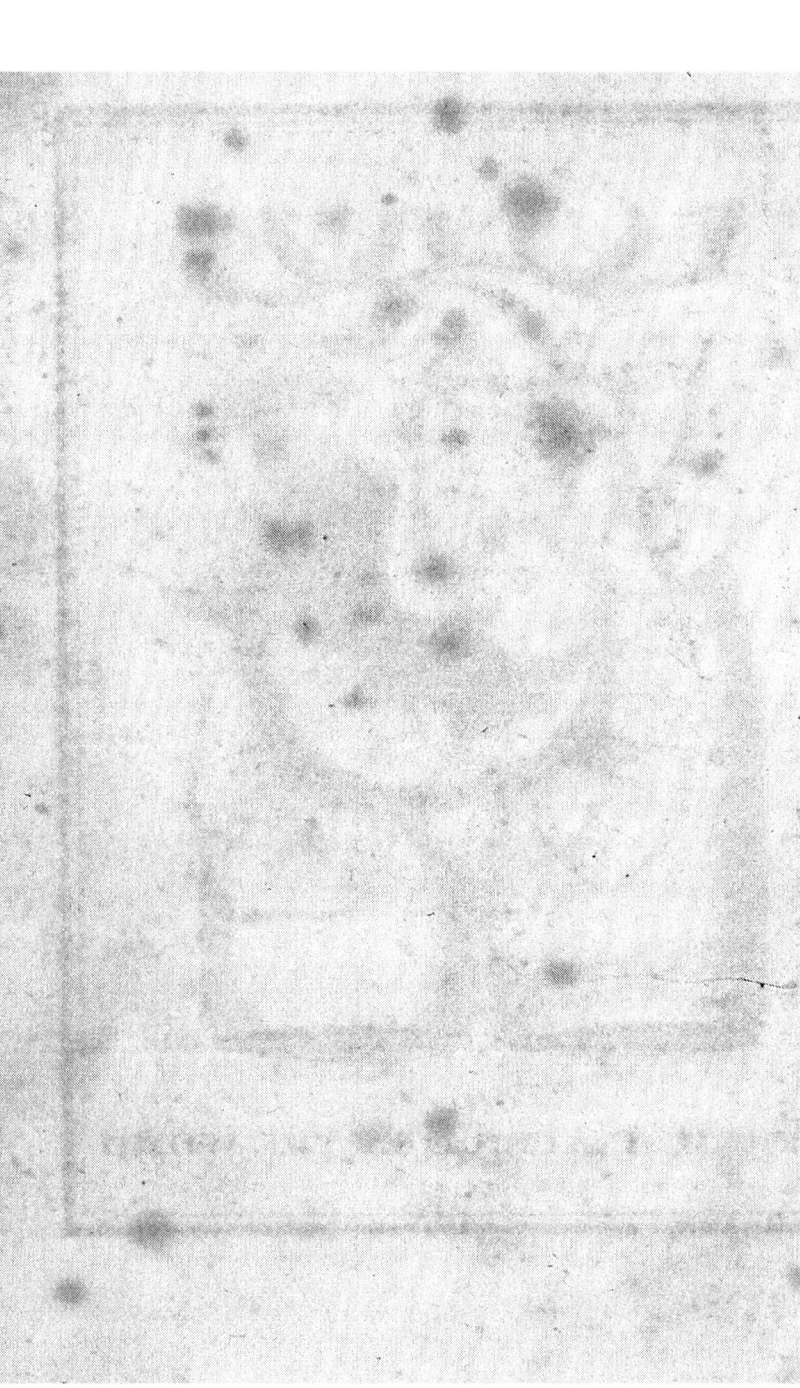

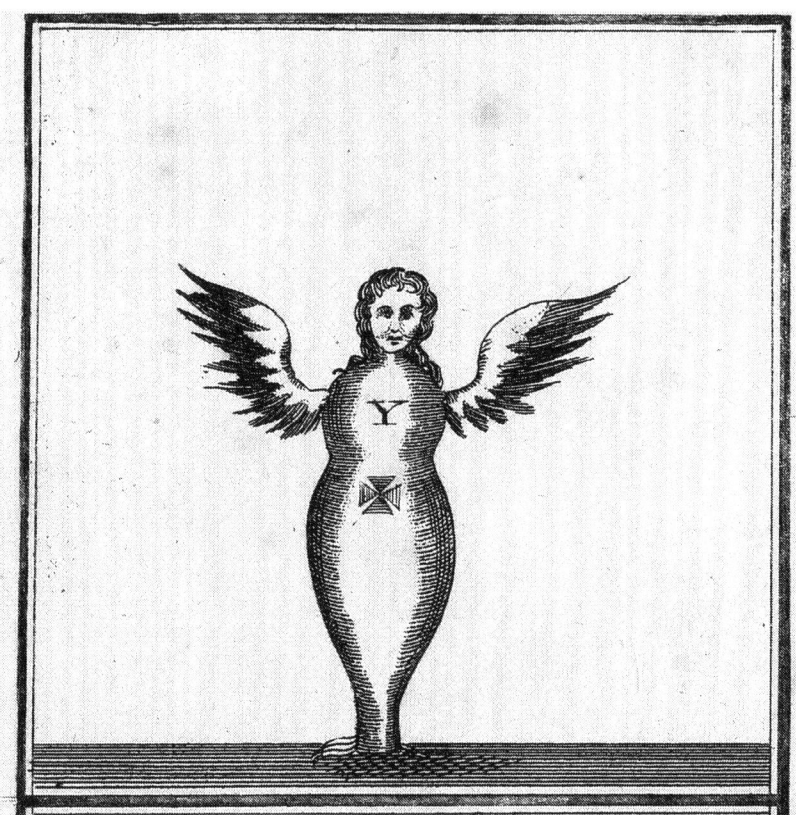

Page 27.

A MONSTER

Like this was born at Ravenna in Italy in the
Year 1512

The matter may be in default two ways—by defect or by excess; by defect, when the child hath but one arm: by excess, when it hath three hands or two heads. Some monsters are begot by a woman's unnatural lying with beasts; as in the year 1603, there was a monster begotten by a woman's generating with a dog: which monster, from the naval upwards, had the perfect resemblance of its mother; but from its naval downwards it resembled a dog, as you may see by the foregoing figure.

The agent, or womb, may be in fault three ways: 1st, The formative faculty, which may be too strong or too weak, by which is procured a depraved figure: 2dly, in the instrument or place of conception: the evil conformation or disposition whereof will cause a monstrous birth: 3dly, In the imaginative power at the time of conception; which is of such a force, that it stamps the character of the thing imagined on the child. So that the children of an adultress may be like her own husband, though begot by another man, which is caused through the force of imagination that the woman hath of her own husband in the act of coition. And I have heard of a woman, who, at the time of conception beholding the picture of a blackamoor, conceived and brought forth an Ethiopian. I will not trouble you with more human testimonies, but conclude with a stronger warrant. We read (Gen. xxx. 31) how Jacob, having agreed with Laban to have all the spotted sheep for keeping his flock, to augment his wages took hazel rods and peeled white strakes on them, and laid them before the sheep when they came to drink, which coupling together there, whilst they beheld the rods, conceived and brought forth young.

Another monster representing an hairy child. It was all covered with hair like a beast. That which rendered it more frightful, was, that its naval was in the place where the nose should stand, and its eyes placed where the mouth should have been: and its mouth was in the chin. It was of the male kind, and was born in France in the year 1597, at a town called Arlest in Province, and lived a few days, frightening all that beheld it. It was looked upon as a forerunner of those desolations which soon after happened in that kingdom, where men towards each other were more like beasts than human creatures.

Likewise, in the reign of Henry III. there was a woman delivered of a child, having two heads and four arms, and the bodies were joined at the backside: the heads were so placed, that they looked contrary ways: each had two distinct arms and hands; they would both laugh, both speak, and both cry, and be hungry together, sometimes the one would speak, and the other would keep silence, and sometimes both speak together. It lived several years, but one outlived the other three years, carrying the dead one (for there was no parting them) till the other fainted with the burden and more with the stink of the dead carcase.

The imagination also works into the child, after conception, for which we have a pregnant instance

A worthy gentlewoman in Suffolk, who being with child, and passing by a butcher killing his meat, a drop of blood sprung on her face; whereupon she said, her child would have a blemish on its face; and at the birth it was found marked with a red spot.

It is certain, that monstrous births often happen by means of undue copulation; for some there are, who having been long absent from one another, and having an eager desire for enjoyment, consider not, as they ought, to do as their circumstances require. And if it happen that they come together when the woman's menses are flowing, and notwithstanding proceed to the act of copulation, which is both unclean and unnatural, the issue of such copulation does often prove monstrous, as a just punishment for doing what nature forbids. And, therefore, though men should be ever so eager for it, yet, women, knowing their own conditions, should at such times refuse their company. And though such copulations do not always produce monstrous births, yet the children, then begotten, are generally heavy, dull, and sluggish, and defective in their understandings, wanting the vivacity and liveliness which children got in proper seasons are endowed with.

By the following figure you may see, that though some of the members may be wanting, yet they are supplied by other members.

It remains now that I make some inquiry, whether those that are born monsters have reasonable souls, and are capable of resurrection. And here both divines and physicians are generally of opinion that those who, according to the order of generation deduced from our first parents, proceed by natural means from either sex, though their outward shape may be deformed and monstrous, have notwithstanding a reasonable soul, and consequently their bodies are capable of a resurrection, as other men's and women's are: but those monsters that are not begotten by men, but are the product of women's unnatural lusts in copulation with other creatures, shall perish as the brute beasts, by whom they were begotten, not having a reasonable soul, or any breath of the Almighty infused into them; and such can never be capable of a resurrection. And the same is also true of imperfect and abortive births.

Some are of opinion, that monsters may be engendered by some infernal spirit. Of this mind was Agidus Facius, speaking of a deformed monster born at Cracovis; and Hironamus Gardanus wrote of a maid that was got with child of a devil, she thinking it had been a fair young man. The like also is recorded by Vicentius, of the prophet Merlin, that he was begotten by an evil spirit. But what a repugnance would it be both to religion and nature, if the devils could beget men; when we are taught to believe, that not any was ever begotten without human seed, except the Son of God: the devil then being a spirit, and having no corporeal substance, has therefore no seed of generation: to say that he can use the act of generation effectually is to affirm, that he can make something of nothing, and consequently to affirm the devil to be God, for creation belongs to God only. Again, if the devil could assume to himself a human body, and enliven the faculties of it, and cause it to generate, as some affirm he can, yet this body must bear the image of the devil. And it borders upon blasphemy to think, that God should so far give leave to the devil, as out of God's image to raise his own diabolical offspring. In the school of nature we are taught the contrary, viz. that like begets like: therefore of a devil cannot man be born. Yet it is not denied, but that devils transforming themselves into human shapes, may abuse both men and women, and with wicked people use carnal copulation; but that any such unnatural conjunction can bring forth a human creature is contrary to nature and religion.

CHAPTER VI.

Of the happy State of Matrimony, as it is appointed by God; the true Felicity that rebounds thereby to either Sex: and to what end it is ordained.

WITHOUT doubt, the uniting of hearts in holy wedlock is of all conditions the happiest; for then a man has a second self to whom he can reveal his thoughts: as well as a sweet companion in his labour: he has one in whose breast, as in a safe cabinet, he may repose his inmost secrets, especially where reciprocal love and inviolate faith is settled. for there no care, fear, jealousy, mistrust, or hatred can ever interpose. For what man ever hated his own flesh?

and truly a wife, if rightly considered, as our grandfather Adam well observed, is or ought to be esteemed of every honest man, "Bone of his bone, and flesh of his flesh," &c. Nor was it the least care of the Almighty to ordain so near a union, and that for two causes; the 1st, for increase of posterity; the 2d, to bridle man's wandering desires and affections: nay, that they might be yet happier, when God had joined them together he "blessed them;" as in Gen. ii. Columila, contemplating this happy state, tells, out of the Economy of Xenophon, that the marriage bed is not only the most pleasant, but profitable course of life, that may be entered on for the preservation and increase of posterity. Wherefore, since marriage is the most safe, sure, and delightful situation of mankind, who is exceeding prone, by the dictates of nature, to propagate his like, he does in no ways provide amis for his own tranquillity who enters into it especially when he comes to maturity of years.

There are many abuses in marriage, contrary to what is ordained, the which, in the ensuing chapter, I shall expose to view. But to proceed: seeing our blessed Saviour and his holy apostles detested unlawful lusts, and pronounced those to be excluded the kingdom of heaven that polluted themselves with adultery and whoring: I cannot conceive what face persons have to colour their impieties, who hating matrimony, make it their study how they may live licentiously; for, in so doing, they rather seek to themselves torment, anxiety, and disquietude, than certain pleasure: besides the hazard of their immortal soul; and certain it is, mercenary love, (or, as the wise man calls it, harlot smiles) cannot be true and sincere, and therefore not pleasant, but rather a net laid to betray such as trust in them into all mischief, as Solomon observes of the young man void of understanding, who turned aside to the harlot's house, "as a bird to the snare of the fowler, or as an ox to the slaughter, till a dart was struck through his liver" Nor in this case can they have children, those endearing affection: or, if they have, they will rather redound to their shame than comfort, bearing the odious brand of bastards. Harlots, likewise, are like swallows, flying in the summer season of prosperity: but the black stormy weather of adversity coming, they take wing and fly into other regions—that is, seek after other lovers; but a virtuous chaste wife, fixing her entire love upon her husband, and submitting to him as her head and king, by whose directions she ought to steer in all lawful courses, will, like a faithful companion, share patiently with him in all adversities, run with cheerfulness through all difficulties and dangers, though ever so hazardous, to preserve or assist him in poverty, sickness, or whatever other misfortunes may befal him, acting according to her duty in all things; but a proud imperious harlot will do no more than she lists, in the sunshine of prosperity; and, like a horse leach, ever craving, and never satisfied; still-seeming displeased, if all her extravagant cravings be not answered; not regarding the ruin and misery which she brings upon him by those means, though she seem to doat upon him, using to confirm her hypocrisy with crocodile tears, vows, and swoonings, when her cully is to depart awhile, or seems but to deny her immoderate desires yet this lusts no longer than she can gratify her appetite, and prey upon his fortune.

Now, on the contrary, a loving, chaste, and even tempered wife, seeks what she may do to prevent such dangers, and in every condition does all to make him easy. And, in a word, as there is no content in the embraces of a harlot, so there is no greater joy than in the reciprocal affection and endearing embraces of a loving, obedient, and chaste wife. Nor is that the principal end for which matrimony was ordained, but that the man might follow the law of his creation, by increasing his kind, and replenishing the earth: for this was the injunction laid upon him in Paradise, before his fall. To conclude, a virtuous wife is a crown and ornament to her husband, and her price is above rubies; but the ways of a harlot are deceitful.

CHAPTER VII.

Of errors in Marriage; Why they are; And the Prejudices of them.

By errors in marriage, I mean the unfitness of the persons marrying to enter into this state, and that both with respect to age, and the constitution of their bodies; and therefore those that design to enter into that condition ought to observe their ability, and not run themselves into inconveniences; for those that marry too young may be said to marry unseasonably, not considering their inability, nor examining the force of nature: for some, before they are ripe for the consummation of so weighty a matter, who either rashly, of their own accord, or by the instigation of procurers, or marriage brokers, or else forced thereto by their parents who covet a large dowry, take upon them this yoke to their prejudice; by which some, before the expiration of a year, have been so enfeebled, that all their vital moisture has been exhausted; which hath not been restored again without great trouble, and the use of medicines. Wherefore, my advice is, that it is no ways convenient to suffer children, or such as are not of age, to marry or get children.

He that proposes to marry, and wishes to enjoy happiness in that state, should choose a wife descended from honest and temperate parents; she being chaste, well bred, and of good manners. For if a woman hath good qualities, she hath portion enough. That of Alcmena, in Plautus, is much to the purpose, where he brings in a young woman speaking thus;

> I take not that to be my dowry, which
>   The vulgar sort do wealth and honour call:
> But all my wishes terminate in this,
>   T' obey my husband, and be chaste withal;
> To have God's fear, and beauty, in my mind,
> To do those good who're virtuously inclin'd.

And I think she was in the right, for such a wife is more precious than rubies.

It is certainly the duty of parents to be careful in bringing up their children in the ways of virtue, and to have regard to their honour and reputation; and especially of virgins, when grown to be marriageable. For, as has been before noted, if through the too much severity of parents, they may be crossed in their love, many of them throw themselves into the unchaste arms of the next alluring tempter that comes in the way, being, through the softness and flexibility of their nature, and the strong desire they have after what nature strongly incites them to, easily induced to believe men's false vows of promised marriage, to cover their shame; and then too late their parents repent of their severity, which has brought an indelible stain upon their families.

Another error in marriage is, the inequality of years in the parties married; such as for a young man who, to advance his fortune, marries a woman old enough to be his grandmother; between whom, for the most part, strife, jealousies, and discontents, are all the blessings which crown the genial bed, it being impossible for such to have any children. The like may be said, though with a little excuse, when an old doting widower marries a virgin in the prime of her youth and vigour, who, while he vainly strives to please her, is thereby wedded to his grave. For as in green youth, it is unfit and unseasonable to think of marriage, so to marry in old age is altogether the same: for they that enter upon it too soon, are soon exhausted, and fall into consumptions and divers other diseases, and those that procrastinate and marry unseemly, fall into the like inconveniences: on the other side having only this honour, if old men they become young cuckolds, especially if their wives have not been trained up in the paths of virtue, and lie too much open to the importunity and temptation of lewd and debauched men. And thus much for the errors of rash and inconsiderate marriages.

CHAPTER VIII.

The Opinion of the Learned concerning Children conceived and born within seven Months; with arguments upon the Subject, to prevent Suspicion of Incontinency, and bitter Contests on that Account. To which are added, Rules to know the Disposition of Man's Body by the Genital Parts.

Many bitter quarrels happen between men and their wives upon the man's supposing that his child comes too soon, and by consequence, that he could not be the father; whereas it is through want of understanding the secrets of nature, that brings the man into that error: and which, had he known might have cured him of his suspicion and jealousy.

To remove which, I shall endeavour to prove, that it is possible, and has been frequently known, that children have been born at seven months. The cases of this nature that have happened have made work for the lawyers, who have left it to the physicians to judge, by viewing the child. whether it be a child of seven, or eight, or ten months Paul. the counsel, has this passage in his 19th Book of Pleadings, viz, "It is now a received truth, that a perfect child may be born in the seventh month, by the authority of the learned Hippocrates: and therefore we must believe, that a child born at the end of the seventh month in lawful matrimony, may be lawfully begotten."

Galen is of opinion, that there is no certain time set for the bearing of children: and that from Pliny's authority, who makes mention of a woman that went 13 months with child; but as to what concerns the 7th month, a learned author says "I know several married people in Holland that had twins born in the 7th month, who lived to old age, having lusty bodies and lively minds. Wherefore their opinion is absurd who assert that a child at 7 months cannot be perfect and long lived; and that it cannot in all parts be perfect till the 9th month. Thereupon this author proceeds to tell a passage from his own knowledge, viz. "Of late there happened a great disturbance among us, which ended not without bloodshed; and was occasioned by a virgin, whose chastity had been violated, descending of a noble family of unspotted fame; several charged the fact upon the judge, who was president of a city in Flanders, who firmly denied it, saying, he was ready to give his oath that he never had any carnal copulation with her, and that he would not father that which was none of his: and farther argued; that he verily believed that it was a child born in 7 months, himself being many miles distant from the mother of it, when it was conceived. Upon which the judges decreed, that the child should be viewed by able physicians and experienced women, and that they should make their report. They having made diligent inquiry, all of them, with one mind, concluded the child without respecting who was the father, was born within the space of 7 months, and that it was carried in the mother's womb but twenty seven weeks and some odd days; but if she should have gone full nine months, the child's parts and limbs would have been more firm and strong, and the structure of the body more compact; for the skin was very loose, and the breast bone that defends the heart, and the gristle that lay over the stomach, lay higher than naturally they should be, not plain, but crooked and sharp, ridged or pointed like those of a young chicken hatched in the beginning of spring.

"And being a female, it wanted nails upon the joints of the fingers; upon which, from the masculous cartilaginous matter of the skin, nails that are very smooth do come, and by degrees harden: she had, instead of nails, a thin skin or film. As for her toes, there was no sign of nails upon them, wanting the heat which was expanded to the fingers from the nearness of the heart. All this being considered, and above all, one gentlewoman of quality that assisted affirming, that she had been the mother of 19 children, and that divers of them had been born and lived at 7 months; they, without favour to any party, made their report, that the infant was a child of 7 months, though within the 7th month: For in such cases, the revolution of the moon ought to be observed, which perfects itself in four bare weeks, or somewhat less than 28 days: in which space of the revolution; the blood being agitated by the force of the moon, the courses of the women flow from them:

which being spent, and the matrix cleansed from the menstruous blood, which happens on the 4th day, then if a man on the 7th day lie with his wife, the copulation is most natural, and then is the conception best: and a child thus begotten may be born in the 7th month and prove very healthful. So that on this report the supposed father was pronounced innocent, on proof that he was 100 miles distant all that month in which the child was begotten: as for the mother, she strongly denied that she knew the father, being forced in the dark; and so through fear and surprise, was left in ignorance."

As for coition, it ought not to be used unless the parties be in health, lest it turn to the disadvantage of the children so begotten, creating in them, through the abundance of ill humours, divers languishing diseases. Wherefore, health is no way better discerned than by the genitals of the man; for which reason midwives, and other skilful women, were formerly wont to see the testicles of children, thereby to conjecture their temperature and state of body: and young men may know thereby the signs or symptoms of death; for if the cases of the testicles be loose and feeble, and the cods fall down, it denotes that the vital spirits, which are the props of life, are fallen; but if the secret parts be wrinkled and raised up it is a sign all is well: but that the event may exactly answer the prediction, it is necessary to consider what part of the body the disease possesseth; for if it chance to be the upper part that is afflicted, as the head or stomach, then it will not so well appear by the members, which are unconcerned with such grievances: but the lower part of the body exactly sympathising with them, their liveliness, or the contrary, makes it apparent; for nature's force, and the spirits that have their intercourse, first manifest themselves therein; which occasions midwives to feel the genitals of children, to know in what part the grief is residing, and whether life or death be portended thereby, the symptoms being strongly communicated to the vessels, that have their intercourse with the principal seat or life.

CHAPTER IX.

Of the Green-sickness in Virgins, with its Causes, Signs, and Cures; together with the chief Occasion of Barrenness in Women, and the Means to remove the Cause, and render them fruitful.

The green-sickness is so common a distemper in virgins, especially those of a phlegmatic complexion, that it is easily discerned, showing itself by discolouring the face, making it look green, pale, and of a dusty colour, proceeding from raw and indigested humours; nor doth it only appear to the eye, but sensibly affects the person with difficulty of breathing, pains in the head, palpitation of the heart, with unusual beatings and small throbbings of the arteries in the temples, neck, and back, which often cast them into fevers, when the humour is overvicious; also loathing of meat, and the distention of the hypocondriac part, by reason of the inordinate effluction of the menstruous blood to the greater vessels: and from the abundance of humours, the whole body is often troubled with swellings, or at least the thighs, legs, and ankles, all above the heels; there is also a great weariness of the body without any reason for it.

The Galenical physicians affirm, that this distemper proceeds from the womb, occasioned by the gross, vicious, and rude humours arising from several inward causes: but there are also outward causes, which have a share in the production of it; as taking cold in the feet, drinking of water, intemperance of diet, eating things contrary to nature, viz. raw or burnt flesh, ashes, coals, old shoes, chalk, wax, nut-shells, mortar, lime, oatmeal, tobacco-pipes, &c. which occasion both a suppression of the menses, and obstructions through the whole body; therefore the first thing necessary to vindicate the cause is matrimonial conjunction, and such copulation as may prove satisfactory to her that is afflicted: for then the menses will begin to flow, according to their natural and due course, and the humours being dispersed will soon waste themselves; and then no more matter being admitted to increase them, they will vanish and a good temperament of body will return; but in case this best remedy cannot be had soon enough, then bleed her in the ankles; and if she be about the age of sixteen, you may likewise do it in the arm; but let her be bled sparingly, especially if the blood be good. If the disease be of any continuance, then it is to be eradicated by purging, preparation of the humour first considered, which may be done by the virgin's drinking the decoction of guiacum, with dittany of Crete; but the best purge in this case ought to be made of aloes, agric, senna, rhubarb: and for strengthening the bowels and opening obstructions, chalybeate medicines are chiefly to be used. The diet must be moderate, and sharp things by all means avoided.

And now since barrenness daily creates discontent, and that discontent breeds difference between man and wife, or, by immediate grief, frequently casts the woman into one or other distemper, I shall in the next place treat thereof.

OF BARRENNESS.

Formerly, before women came to the marriage-bed, they were first searched by the midwife, and those only which she allowed of as fruitful were admitted. I hope, therefore, it will not be amiss to show you how they may prove themselves, and turn barren ground into a fruitful soil. Barrenness is a deprivation of the life and power which ought to be in seed to procreate and propagate; for which end men and women were made. Causes of barrenness may be overmuch cold or heat, drying up the seed, and corrupting it, which extinguishes the life of the seed, making it waterish and unfit for generation. It may be caused also by the not flowing or overflowing of the courses; by swelling, ulcers, and inflamations of the womb, by an excrescence of flesh growing about the mouth of the matrix, by the mouth of the matrix being turned to the back or side, by the fatness of the body, whereby the mouth of the matrix is closed up, being pressed with the omentum or caul, and the matter of the seed is turned to fat; if she be of a lean and dry body, and though she do conceive, yet the fruit of her body will wither before it come to perfection, for want of nourishment. One main cause of barrenness is attributed to want of a convenient moderating quality, which the woman ought to have with the man; as if he be hot, she must be cold: if he be dry, she must be moist; but if they be both dry or both moist of constitution, they cannot propagate; and yet, simply considered of themselves, they are not barren; for he and she who were before as the barren fig-tree, being joined to an apt constitution, become as the fruitful vine. And that a man and woman being every way of like constitution cannot procreate, I will bring nature itself for a testimony; who hath made man of the better constitution than woman, that the quality of the one may moderate the quality of the other.

Signs of Barrenness. If barrenness doth proceed from overmuch heat, she is of dry body, subject to anger, hath black hair, quick pulse, her purgations flow but little, and that with pain, and she loves to play in the courts of Venus. But if it comes by cold, then are the signs contrary to these above mentioned. If through the evil quality of the womb, make a suffumigation of red storax. myrrh, cassia wood, nutmeg, and cinnamon: and let her receive the fume of it into the womb, covering her very close: and if the odour so received passeth through the body to the mouth and nostrils. she is fruitful. But if she feels not the fume in her mouth and nose, it argues barrenness one of these ways—that the spirit of the seed is either through cold extinguished, or through heat dissipated. If any woman be suspected to be unfruitful. cast natural brimstone, such as is digged out of the mine, into her urine; and if worms breed therein, she is not barren.

Prognostics. Barrenness makes women look young, because they are free from those pains and sorrows which other women are accustomed to. Yet they have not the full perfection of health which fruitful women do enjoy, because they are not rightly purged of the menstruous blood and superfluous seed, which are the principal causes of most uterine diseases.

Cure. First, the cause must be removed, the womb strengthened, and the spirits of the seed enlivened.

If the womb be over-hot, take syrup of succory, with rhubarb, syrup of violets. endive, roses, cassia, purslain. Take of endive, water-lilies, borage flowers, of each a handful; rhubarb, mirobalans, of each three drams: with water make a decoction: and to the straining of the syrup add electuary of violets one ounce, syrup of cassia half an ounce, manna three drams; make a potion. Take of syrup of mugwort one ounce, syrup of maiden-hair two ounces. pulv. elect. trias and one dram; make a julep. Take prus. salt. elect. ros. mesua, of each three drams. rhubarb one scruple, and make a bolus; apply to the reins and privities fomentations of the juice of lettuce, violets, roses, malloes. vine leaves. and night-shade; anoint the secret parts with the cooling unguent of Galen.

If the power of the seed be extinguished by cold, take every morning two spoonfuls of cinnamon water, with one scruple of mithridate. Take syrup of calamint, mugmort. and betony, of each one ounce: water of penny-royal. feverfew, hyssop, and sage, of each two ounces: make a julep. Take oil of anniseed two scruples and a half; diacimini, diacilathidi-

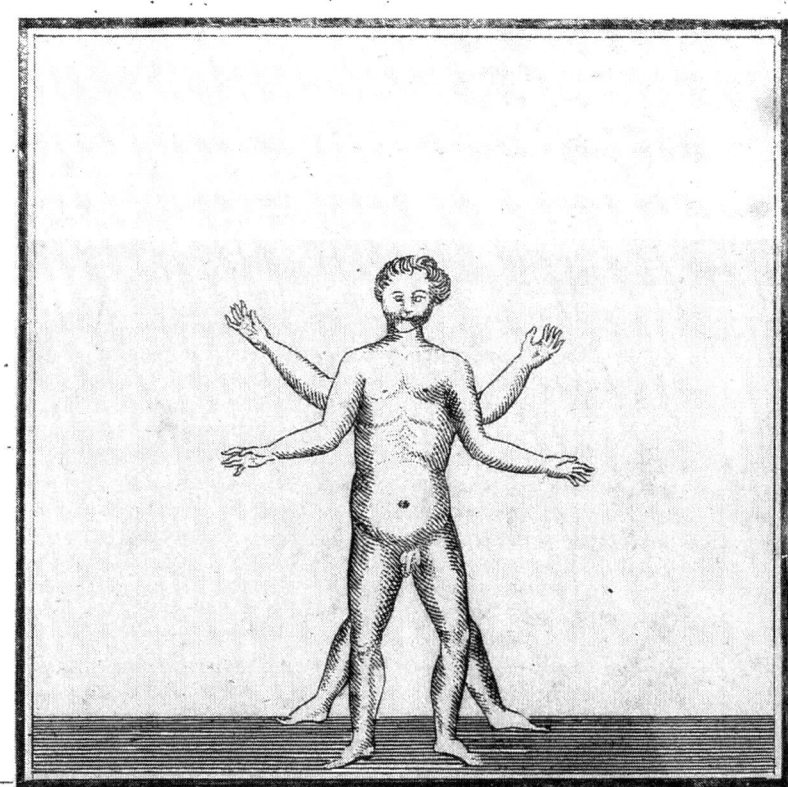

Page 28.

A MONSTER

Like this was born at Nazara, in the Year 1530
It had four arms and four legs.

amosei, and diagla-angae, of each one oram, sugar four ounces, with water of cinnamon, and make lozenges; take of them a dram and a half twice a-day, two hours before meals; fasten cupping-glasses to the hips and belly. Take of storax and calamint one ounce, mastich, cinnamon, nutmeg, lign, aloes and frankincense, of each half an ounce; musk ten grains, ambergrease half a scruple: with rose-water make a confection, divide it into four equal parts; of one part make a pomum oderatum, to smell to, if she be not hysterical; of the second make a mass of pills, and let her take three every night; of the third make a pessary, dip it in the oil of spikenard, and put it up; of the fourth make a suffumigation for the womb.

If the faculties of the womb be weakened, and the life of the seed suffocated by over much humidity flowing to those parts: take of betony, marjoram, mugwort, penny-royal, and balm, of each a handful; roots of allom and fennel, of each two drams; anniseed and cummin, of each one dram, with sugar and water a sufficient quantity; make a syrup, and take three ounces every morning.

Purge with the following things: take of the diagnidium two grains, specierum of castor a scruple, pillfœdit two scruples, with syrup of mugwort; make six pills. Take specdiagem, diamoser, diamb. of each one dram; cinnamon one dram and a half; cloves, mace and nutmeg, of each half a dram; sugar six ounces, with water of feverfew: make lozenges, to be taken every morning. Take of the decoction of salsaporilla, and virga-aurea, not forgetting sage, which Agrippa, wondering at its operation, hath honoured with the name of sacra herba, a holy herb, and is recorded by Dodonæus in the History of Plants, lib. ii. cap. 77: that after a great mortality among the Egyptians, the surviving women, that they might multiply quickly, were commanded to drink the juice of sage, anoint the genitals with oil of anniseed and spikenard. Take mace, nutmeg, cinnamon, storax and amber, of each one dram; cloves, laudanum, of each half a dram: turpentine, a sufficient quantity; trochisks, to smooth the womb. Take roots of valerian and elecampane, of each one pound; galanga, two ounces: origan, lavender, marjoram, betony, mugwort, bay-leaves, calamint, of each a handful; with water make an infusion, in which let her sit, after she hath her courses.

If barrenness proceed from dryness, consuming the matter of the seed, take every day almond milk, and goat's milk extracted with honey: but often of the root satyon candied, and of the electuary of diasyren. Take three wethers' heads, boil them till all the flesh come from the bones; then take melilot, violets, camomile, mercury, orchia with their roots, of each a handful: fenugreek, linseed, valerian roots, of each one pound; let all these be decocted in the aforesaid broth, and let the woman sit in the decoction up to the navel.

If barrenness be caused by any proper effect of the womb the cure is set down in the second part. Sometimes the womb proves barren where there is no impediment on either side, except only in the manner of the act; as when in the emission of the seed, the man is quick, and the woman too slow, whereby there is not an emission of both seeds at the same instant, as the rules of conception require. Before the acts of coition, foment the private parts with the decoction of betony, sage, hyssop, and calamint, and anoint the mouth and neck of the womb with musk and civet.

The cause of barrenness being removed, let the womb be corroborated as follows. Take of bayberries, mastic, nutmeg, frankincense, nuts, laudanum, giapanum, of each one dram, styracis liquid, two scruples, cloves, half a scruple, ambergrease, two grains, then with oil of spikenard make a pessary.

Take of red roses, lapidis hæmatis, white frankincense, of each half an ounce. Sanguis draconis, fine bole, mastic, of each two drams; nutmeg, cloves, of each one dram; spikenard half a scruple; with oil of wormwood; make a plaister for the lower part of the belly: then suffer her to eat often of eringo roots candied: and make an injection only of the roots of satyrion.

The aptest time for conception is instantly after the menses are ceased, because then the womb is thirsty and dry, apt both to draw the seed, and return it, by the roughness of the inward superfices. And, besides, in some, the mouth of the womb is turned into the back or side, and is not placed right until the last day of the courses.

Excess in all things is to be avoided. Lay aside all passions of the mind; shun study and care, as things that are enemies to conception: for, if a woman conceive under such circumstances, how wise soever the parents are, the children at best will be but foolish: because the mental faculties of the parent, viz. the understanding and the rest (from whence the child derives its reason) are, as it were, confused through the multiplicity of cares and cogitations: examples hereof we have in learned men, who, after great study and care, accompanying with their wives, very often beget very foolish children. A hot and moist air is most convenient, as appears by the women of Egypt, who usually bring forth three or four children at one time.

CHAPTER X.

Virginity, what it is, in what it consists, and how vitiated; together with the Opinion of the Learned about the Mutation of the Sex in the Womb, during the Operation of Nature in forming the Body.

THERE are many ignorant people that boast of their skill in the knowledge of virginity, and some virgins have undergone hard censures through their ignorant determinations; and, therefore, I thought it highly necessary to clear this point, that the towering imaginations of conceited ignorance may be brought down, and the fair sex (whose virtues are so illustriously bright, that they excite our wonder, and command our imitation) may be freed from the calumnies and detractions of ignorance and envy; and so their honours may continue as unspotted as they have kept their persons uncontaminated and free of defilement.

Virginity, in a strict sense, does signify the prime, the chief, the best of any thing, which makes men so desirous of marrying virgins, imagining some secret pleasure to be enjoyed in their embraces, more than in those of widows, or such as have been lain withal: though not many years ago, a very great person was of another mind; and, to use his own expression,—"That the getting of a maidenhead was such a piece of drudgery, as was more proper for a porter than a prince." But this was only his opinion, for most men, I am sure, have other sentiments. But to return to our purpose.

The curious inquirers into nature's secrets have observed, that in young maids in the sinus pudoris, or in that place which is called the neck of the womb, is that wondrous production, vulgarly called the hymen, but more rightly the claustrum virginale; and in the French, bouton de rose, or rose-bud: because it resembles the bud of a rose expanded, or a convex gillyflower. From hence is derived the word defloro, or deflower; and hence taking away virginity is called deflowering a virgin; most being of opinion, that the virginity is altogether lost, when this duplication is fractured and dissipated by violence; and when it is found perfect and entire, no penetration has been made; and it is the opinion of some learned physicians, that there is neither hymen, nor skin expanded containing blood in it, which divers think, in the first copulation, flows from the fractured expanse.

Now this claustrum, or virginale, or flower, is composed of four carbuncles, or little buds like myrtle berries, which, in virgins, are full and plump, but in women flag and hang loose; and these are placed in the four angles of the sinus pudoris, joined together by little membranes and ligatures like fibres, each of them situated in the testicles, or spaces between each carbuncle, with which, in a manner, they are proportionally distended; which membranes being once delacerated denote devirgination; and many inquisitive, and yet ignorant persons, finding their wives defective therein the first not of their marriage, have thereupon suspected their chastity, and concluded another had been there before them. Now to undeceive such, I do affirm, that such fractures happen divers accidental ways, as well as by copulation with men, viz. by violent straining, coughing, sneezing, stopping of urine, and violent motions of the vessels, forcibly sending down the humours, which, pressing for passage, break the ligatures or membrane: so that the fracture of that which is commonly taken for their virginity, or maidenhead, is no absolute sign of dishonesty: though certain it is, that it broke in copulation oftener than by any other means.

I have heard, that at an assize held at Rutland, a young man was tried for a rape, in forcing a virgin; when, after divers questions being asked, and the maid swearing positively to the matter naming the time, place, and manner of the action; it was upon mature deliberation resolved, that she should be searched by a skilful surgeon and two midwifes, who were to make their report upon oath; which, after due examination, they accordingly did, affirming that the membranes were entire, and not delacerated: and that it was their opinion, for that reason, that her body had not been penetrated: which so far wrought with the jury, that the prisoner was acquitted; and the maid afterwards confessed, she swore against him out of revenge, he having promised to marry her, and afterwards declined it. And thus much shall suffice to be spoken concerning virginity.

I shall now proceed to something of nature's operation, in mutation of sexes in the womb.

This point is of much necessity, by reason of the different opinions of men relating to it; therefore, before any thing positively can be asserted, it will be proper to recite what has been delivered, as well in the negative as affirmative. And first, Severus Plinus, who argues for the negative, writes thus: The genital parts of both sexes are so unlike each other in substance, composition, situation, figure, action, and use, that nothing is more unlike, and by how much more all parts of the body (the breasts excepted, which in women swell more, because nature ordained them for suckling the infant) have exact resemblance, so much more do the genital parts of the one sex, compared with the other, differ: and if their figure be thus different, much more their use. The venereal appetite also proceeds from different causes: for in a man it proceeds from a desire of emission, and in woman from a desire of reception; in women also the chief of these parts are concave and apt to receive; but in men they are more porous. All these things being considered, I cannot but wonder, says he, how any one can imagine that the genital members of the female births should be changed into those that belong to the male, since by those parts only the distinction of the sexes is made; nor can I well impute the reason of this vulgar error to any thing but the mistake of inexpert midwifes, who have been deceived by the evil conformation of the parts, which, in some male births, may have happened to have some small protusions, not to have been discerned, as appears by the example of a child, christened at Paris by the name of Joan, as a girl, who afterwards proved a boy: and, on the contrary, the over-far extension of the clytoris in female-births may have occasioned the like mistakes. Thus far Pliny proceeds in the negative: and yet, notwithstanding what he hath said, there are divers learned physicians that have asserted the affirmative, of which number Galen is one. A man, saith he, is different from a woman is nothing else but having his genital members without his body, whereas a woman has them within. And this is certain, that if nature, having formed a male should convert him into a female, she hath no other task to perform, but to turn his genital members inward: and so to turn a woman into a man by the contrary operation. But this is to be understood of the child, when it is in the womb, and not perfectly formed; for, oft-times, nature hath made a female child, and it hath so remained in the womb of the mother for a month or two; and after plenty of heat increasing in the genital members, they have issued forth, and the child has become a male, yet retaining some certain gestures unbefitting the masculine sex, as female actions, a shrill voice, and a more effeminate temper than ordinary; contrarywise, nature having often made a male, and cold humours flowing to it, the genitals have been inverted, yet still retaining a masculine air, both in voice and gestures. Now, though both these opinions are supported by several seasons, yet I esteem the latter more agreeable to truth; for there is not that vast difference between the genitals of the two sexes, as Pliny would have us believe there is; for a woman has in a manner the same members with the man, though they appear not outward, but are inverted for the conveniency of generation; the chief difference being, that the one is solid and the other porous, and that the principal reason for changing sexes is, and must be attributed to, heat or cold, suddenly or slowly contracted, which operates according to its greater or lesser force.

CHAPTER XI.

Directions and Cautions for Midwifes: and first how a Midwife ought to be qualified.

A MIDWIFE that would acquit herself well in her employment, ought by no means to enter upon it rashly or unadvisedly, but with all imaginable caution, considering that she is accountable for all the mischief that befalls the female through her wilful ignorance or neglect. Therefore let none take upon them the office barely upon pretence of maturity of years and child bearing, for in such, for the most part, there are divers things wanting that ought to be observed, which is the occasion so many women and children are lost.

Now, for a midwife, in relation to her person, these things ought to be observed, viz.—She must neither be too old nor too young; neither extraordinarily fat nor weakened by leanness, but in a good habit of body: nor subject to diseases fears, and sudden frights; her body well shaped, and neat in her attire; her hands smooth and small, her nails ever paired short, not suffering any rings to be upon her fingers during the time she is doing her office, nor any thing upon her wrists that may obstruct. And to these ought to be added activity and a convenient strength, with much cautiousness and diligence, nor subject to drowsiness, nor apt to be impatient.

As for her manners, she ought to be courteous, affable, sober, chaste, and not subject to passion, bountiful and compassionate to the poor, and not covetous when she attends upon the rich.

Her temper should be cheerful and pleasant, that she may the better comfort her patient in her labours. Nor must she at any time make overmuch haste, though her business should require her in another case, lest she thereby endanger the mother or the child.

Of spirit, she ought to be wary, prudent, and cunning; but, above all, the fear of God ought to have the ascendant in her soul, which will give her both "knowledge and discretion," as the wise man tells us.

CHAPTER XII.

Further Directions for Midwives, teaching them what they ought to do, and what to avoid.

Since the office of a midwife has so great an influence on the well or ill-doing of women and children, in the first place, let her be diligent to acquire whatever knowledge may be advantageous to her practice; never thinking herself so perfect, but that she may add to her knowledge by study and experience; yet never let her make any experiment which may prove distressful to her patient, nor apply any unless she has tried them before, or knows they will do no harm: imposing neither upon poor nor rich, but speaking freely what she knows; and by no means prescribing such medicines as will cause abortion, though desired: which is a high degree of wickedness, and may be termed murder. If she be sent for to one she knows not, let her be very cautious ere she goes, lest, by laying an infectious woman, she do injury to others, as sometimes it has happened. Neither must she make her house a receptacle for great bellied women to discharge their burdens in, lest her house get an ill name, and she thereby suffer loss.

In laying of women, if the birth happen to be large and difficult, she must not seem to be concerned, but must cheer up the woman, and do what she can to make her labor easy. For which she may find directions in the second part of this book.

She must never think of any thing but doing well, causing all things to be in readiness that are proper for the work, and the strengthening of the woman, and receiving of the child; and, above all, let her take care to keep the woman from being unruly when her throes are coming upon her, lest she thereby endanger her own life and the child's.

She must also take care that she be not too hasty in her business, but wait God's time for the birth; lest, through fear, if things should not go well, it should make her incapable of giving that assistance which the labouring woman stands in need of; for when there is most seeming danger, there is most need of prudence to set things right.

And now, because she can never be a skilful midwife that knows nothing but what is to be seen outwardly. I think it will not be amiss, but on the contrary highly necessary, with modesty, to describe the generative parts of women, as they have been anatomized by the learned, and show the use of such vessels as contribute to generation.

CHAPTER XIII.

Of the Genitals of Women, external and internal, to the Vessels of the Womb.

IF it were not for public benefit, especially of the practitioners and professors of the art of midwifery, I would forbear to treat of the secrets of nature, because they may be turned by some into ridicule: but, being absolutely necessary to be known, I will not omit them. Those parts exposed at the bottom of the belly are the fissura magna, or the great chink, with its labia or lips, the Mons Veneris, and the hair; these are called the pudenda, because, when bare, they bring pudor, or shame, upon a woman. The fissura magna reaches from the lower part of the os pubis to within an inch of the anus; but it is lesser and closer in maids than in those that have borne children, and has two lips, which, towards the pubis, grow thicker and more full; and meeting upon the middle of the os pubis, make that rising hill called Mons Veneris, or the Hill of Venus. Next are the nympha and clytoris; the former is of a membrany and flammy substance, spungy, soft, and partly fleshy, of a red colour, in the shape of wings, two in number, though, from their rise, they are joined in an acute angle, producing there a fleshy substance, which clothes the clytoris: and sometimes they spread so far, that incision is required to make way for the man's instrument of generation.

The clytoris is a substance in the upper part of the division where the two wings concur, and is the seat of venereal pleasure, being like a yard in situation, substance, composition, and erection; growing sometimes out of the body two inches; but that never happens unless through extreme lust or extraordinary accidents. This clytoris consists of two spungy and skinny bodies, containing a distinct original from the os pubis, the head of it being covered with a tender skin, having a hole or passage like the penis or yard of a man, though not quite through, in which, and the bigness, it only differs from it.

The next things are the fly-knobs, and the great neck of the womb. Those knobs are behind the wings, being four in number, and resemble myrtle-berries, being placed quadrangularly; one against the other; and in this place is inserted the orifice of the bladder, which opens itself into the fissures, to evacuate the urine; for securing of which from cold, or the like inconveniency, one of these knobs is placed before it, and shuts up the passage.

The lips of the womb, that next appear, being separated, disclose the neck thereof; and in them two things are to be observed, which is the neck itself, and the hymen, but more properly the claustrum virginale, of which before I have discoursed. By the neck of the womb is to be understood the channel that is between the aforesaid knobs and the inner bone of the womb, which receives the penis like a sheath; and that it may be the better dilated from the pleasure of procreation, the substance of it is sinewy and a little spungy; and in this concavity are divers folds, or obicular plaits, made by tunicles wrinkled like an expanded roset. In virgins they plainly appear, but in women that have often used copulation they are extinguished, so that the inner side of the womb's neck appears smooth, but in old women it appears more hard and gristled. But though this channel be sometimes writhed and crooked, sinking down, yet, in the time of copulation, labour, or the monthly purgation, it is erected and extended; which overtension occasions the pain in child-birth.

The hymen, or claustrum virginale, is that which closes the neck of the womb, being broken in first copulation, its use being rather to stay the untimely courses in virgins than to any other end; and commonly when broken in copulation, or by any other accident, a small quantity of blood flows from it, attended with some little pain. From whence some observe, that between the duplicity of the two tunicles, which constitute the neck of the womb, there are many veins and arteries running along and arising from the vessels on both sides of the thigh, and so passing into the neck of the womb, being very large; and the reason thereof is, that the neck of the bladder requires to be filled with abundance of spirits, thereby to be dilated, for its better taking hold of the penis, there being great heat required in such motions, which becomes more intense by the act of friction, and consumes a considerable quantity of moisture, in the supply of which, large vessels are altogether necessary.

Another cause of the largeness of these vessels is, by reason the menses make their way threw them, which often occasions women with child to continue their purgation, for, though the womb be shut up, yet the neck in the passage of the womb, through which these vessels pass, are open. In this case there is further to be observed, that as soon as you penetrate the pudendum, there appear two little pits or holes, wherein is contained humour, which being expunged in time of copulation, greatly delights the woman.

CHAPTER XIV.

A Description of the Woman's Fabric, the Preparing Vessels and Testicles in Women. As also of the Difference and Ejaculatory Vessels.

In the lower part of the hypogastrium, where the lips are widest and broadest, they being greater and broader thereabout than those of men, for which reason they have likewise broader buttocks than men; the womb is joined to its neck, and is placed between the bladder and straightgut, which keep it from swaying or rolling, yet give it liberty to stretch and dilate itself, and again to contract, as nature disposeth it. Its figure is in a manner round, and not unlike a gourd lessening a little, and growing more accute towards one end, being knit together by its proper ligaments: its neck likewise is joined by its own substance and certain membranes that fasten unto the os sacrum and the share-bone. As to its largeness, that much differs in women, especially the difference is great between those that have borne children, and those that have borne none; in substance it is so thick that it exceeds a thimble-breadth; which, after copulation, is so far from decreasing, that it augments to a greater proportion; and the more to strengthen it, it is interwoven with fibres overthwart, which are both strait and winding: and its proper vessels are veins, arteries, and nerves; and among these there are two little veins, which pass from the spermatic vessels into the bottom of the womb, and two larger from the neck, the mouth of these veins piercing as far as the inward concavity.

The womb hath two arteries on both sides of the spermatic vessels and the hypogastric, which accompany the veins; and besides, there are divers little nerves, that are knit and twined in the form of a net, which are also extended throughout, even from the bottom of the pudendum itself, being placed chiefly for sense and pleasure, moving in sympathy between the head and the womb.

Now, it is to be further noted, that by reason of the two ligaments that hang on either side of the womb, from the share-bone, piercing through the peritoneum, and joined to the bone itself, the womb is moveable upon sundry occasions, often falling low or rising high. As for the neck of the womb, it is of exquisite feeling: so that if it be at any time out of order, being troubled with a schirrosity, over fatness, moisture, or relaxation, the womb is subjected thereby to barrenness. In those that are with child, there frequently stays a glutinous matter in the entrance to facilitate the birth; for, at the time of delivery, the mouth of the womb is opened to such a wideness as is conformable to the bigness of the child, suffering an equal dilation from the bottom to the top.

As for the preparatory, or spermatic vessels, in women, they consist of two veins and two arteries, not differing from those of men, but only in their largeness and manner of insertion: for the number of veins and arteries is the same as in men, the right vein issuing from the trunk of the hollow vein descending; and beside them are two arteries, which flow from the aorta.

As to the length and breadth of these vessels, they are narrower and shorter in women than in men: only, observe, they are more writhed and contorted than in men, and shrinking together, by reason of their shortness, that they may, by their looseness, be better stretched out when occasion requires it; and those vessels in women are carried in an indirect course through the lesser guts and testicles, but are mid-way divided into two branches: the greater goes to the stones, constituting a various or winding body, and wonderfully inoculating: the lesser branch ending in the womb, in the inside of which it disperseth itself, and especially at the higher part of the bottom of the womb, for its nourishment, and that part of the courses may purge through the vessels: and seeing the testicles of women are seated near the womb, for that cause these vessels fall not from the peritoneum, neither make they much passage, as in men, not extending themselves in the share-bone.

The stones in women, commonly called testicles, perform not the same action as in men; they are also different in their location, bigness, temperature, substance, form, and covering. As for the place of their seat, it is in the hollowness of the abdomen; neither are they pendulous, but rest on the muscles of the loins, so that they may, by contracting the greater heat, be more fruitful, their office being to contain the ova, or eggs, one of which being impregnated by the man's seed engenders man; yet they differ from those of men in figure, by reason of their lessness or flatness at each end, not being so round or oval: the external superfices being likewise more unequal, appearing like the composition of a great many knobs or kernels mixed together. There is a difference also in their substance, they being much more soft and pliable, loose, and not so well compacted. Their bigness and temperament are likewise different; for they are much colder, and less than those in men. As for their covering or enclosure, it differs extremely; for as men's are wrapped in divers unicles, by reason they are extremely pendulous, and subject to divers injuries, unless so fenced by nature; so women's stones, being internal, and less subject to casuality, are covered with one tunicle or membrane, which, though it closely cleave to them, yet they are likewise half covered with the peritoneum.

The ejaculatory vessels are two obscure passages, one on each side, nothing differing from the spermatic veins in substance. They rise in one part from the bottom of the womb, not reaching from the other extremity, either to the stones or to any other part, but shut up and impassable, adhering to the womb, as the colon does to the blind gut, and winding half way about; and though the testicles are remote from them, and touch them not, yet they are tied to them by certain membranes, resembling the wing of a bat, through which certain veins and arteries passing from the end of the testicles, may be termed here to have their passage proceeding from the corner of the womb to the testicles, and are accounted proper ligaments, by which the testicles and womb are united and strongly knit together; and these ligaments in women are the cremasters in men, of which I shall speak more largely when I come to describe the masculine parts conducing to generation.

CHAPTER XV.

A Description of the Use and Action of several Parts in Women, appointed in Generation.

The externals, commonly called the pudenda, are designed to cover the great orifice, and to receive the penis or yard in the act of coition, and give passage to the birth and urine. The use of the wings and knobs, like myrtle-berries, are for the security of the internal parts, shutting the orifice and neck of the bladder, and by their swelling up, to cause titilation and delight in those parts, and also to obstruct the involuntary passage of the urine.

The action of the clytoris in women is like that of the penis in man, viz. the erection; and its outer end is like the glands of the penis, and has the same name. And as the glands of man are the seat of the greatest pleasure in conception, so is this in the woman.

The action and use of the neck of the womb is equal with that of the penis, viz. erection, occasioned divers ways: first, in copulation, it is erected and made strait for the passage of the penis into the womb; 2dly, whilst the passage is repleted with spirit and vital blood, it becomes more strait for embracing the penis; and as for the conveniency of erection, it is twofold: first, because if the neck of the womb was not erected, the yard could have no convenient passage to the womb: secondly, it hinders any hurt or damage that might ensue through the violent concussion of the yard during the time of copulation.

As for the veins that pass through the neck of the womb, their use is to replenish it with blood and spirit, that still, as the moisture consumes by the heat contracted in copulation, it may by these vessels be renewed; but their chief business is to convey nutriment to the womb.

The womb has many properties attributed to it: as, first, retention of the fœcundated egg, and this is properly called conception: secondly, to cherish and nourish it, till nature has framed the child and brought it to perfection, and then it strongly operates in sending forth the birth, when the time

E

of its remaining there is expired, dilating itself in a wonderful manner, and so aptly removed from the senses, that nothing of injury can proceed from thence, retaining itself a power and strength to operate and cast forth the birth, unless by accident it be rendered deficient; and then, to strengthen and enable it, remedies must be applied by skilful hands; directions for applying of which will be given in the second part.

The use of the preparing vessels is this: the arteries convey the blood to the testicles; part whereof is put in the nourishment of them, and the production of these little bladders (in all things resembling eggs,) through which the vast preparentia run, and are obliterated in them: and as for the veins, their office is to bring back what blood remains from the use aforesaid. The vessels of this kind are much shorter in women than in men, by reason of their nearness to the stones: which defects are yet made good by the many intricate windings to which those vessels are subject: for, in the middle way they divide themselves into two branches, though different in magnitude, for one being greater than the other, passes to the stones.

The stones in women are very useful, for where they are defective, generation-work is at an end. For although those bladders which are on their outward superfices contain nothing of seed, as the followers of Galen and Hippocrates did erroneously imagine, yet they contain several eggs, generally twenty in each testicle: one of which being impregnated by the spirituous part of the man's seed in the act of coition, descends through the ovaducts into the womb, and from hence, in process of time, becomes a living child.

CHAPTER XVI.

Of the Organs of Generation in Man.

Having given you a description of the organs of generation in women, with the anatomy of the fabric of the womb, I shall now, to complete the first part of this treatise, describe the organs of generation in men, and how they are fitted to the use for which nature designed them.

The instrument of generation in man (commonly called the

yard, and in Latin, penis, a pendendo, because it hangs without the belly,) is an organical part, which consists of skin, tendons, veins, arteries, sinews, and great ligaments; and is long and round, and on the upper side flattish, seated under the os pubis, and ordained by nature partly for evacuation of urine, and partly for conveying the seed into the matrix: for which end it is full of small pores, through which the seed passes into it, through the vesiculæ seminales, and also the neck of the vesiculæ urinalis, which pours out the urine when they make water; besides the common parts, viz. the two nervous bodies, the septum, the urethra, the glands, four muscles, and the vessel. The nervous bodies (so called,) are surrounded with a thick white pervious membrane, but their inmost substance is spungy, consisting chiefly of veins, arteries, and nervous fibres, interwoven together like a net. And when the nerves are filled with animal spirits, and the arteries with hot and spirituous blood, then the penis is distended, and becomes erect; but when the influx of the spirits ceases, then the blood and remaining spirits are absorbed by the veins, and so the penis' spirits are limber and flaggy. Below these nervous bodies is the urethra; and whenever the nervous bodies swell, it swells also. The muscles of the penis are four; two shorter, arising from the coxendix, and serving for erection, and for that reason are called erectores; two larger, proceeding from the spinchter of the anus, which serve to dilate the urethra for evacuation of seed, and are called dilatantes or winding. At the end of the penis are the glands, covered with a very thin membrane, by means of which, and its nervous substance, it becomes most exquisitely sensible, and is the principal seat of pleasure in copulation. The outmost covering of the glands is called præputium, a percutiendo, from being cut off, it being that which the Jews cut off in circumcision, and it is tied by the lower parts of it to the glands of the fœtus. The penis is also stocked with veins, arteries, and nerves.

The testiculi, or stones, (so called, because testifying one to be a man,) elaborate the blood brought to them by the spermatic arteries into seed. They have coats of two sorts, proper and common: the common are two, and invest both the testes. The outermost of the common coats consists of the cuticula, or true skin, and is called the scrotum, hanging out of the abdomen like a purse: the innermost is the membrana carnosa. The proper coats are also two, the outer called cliotrodes or virginales, the inner albugidia: into the outer is inserted the cremaster. To the upper part of the testes are fixed the epidimydes, or prostratæ; from whence ariseth the vasa deferentia, or ejaculatoria; which, when they come near the neck of the bladder, deposit the seed into the vesiculæ seminales, these vesiculæ seminales are two, each like a bunch of grapes, and emit the seed into the urethra in the act of copulation. Near them are the prostatæ, about the bigness of a walnut, and join to the neck of the bladder. Authors do not agree about the use of them, but most are of opinion that they afford an oily, sloppy, and fat humour, to besmear the urethra: whereby to defend the same from the acrimony of the seed and urine. But the vessels which convey the blood to the testes, out of which the seed is made, are arteriae spermaticae, and are also two. The veins which carry out the remaining blood are two, and have the name venae spermaticae.

CHAPTER XVII.

A Word of Advice to both Sexes, being several Directions respecting the Act of Copulation.

Since nature has implanted in every creature a mutual desire of copulation, for the increase and propigation of the kind, and more especially in man, the lord of the creation and master-piece of nature, that so noble a piece of divine workmanship might not perish, something ought to be said concerning it, it being the foundation of all that we have hitherto been treating of, since without copulation there can be no generation. Seeing therefore so much depends upon it, I thought it necessary, before I concluded the first part, to give directions to both sexes, for the performance of that act, as may appear efficacious to the end for which nature designed it: but it will be done with caution as not to offend the chastest ear, nor put the fair sex to the trouble of a blush in reading it. First, then, when a married couple, form a desire of having children, are about to make use of those means that nature ordained to that purpose, it would be very proper to cherish the body with generous restoratives, that so it may be brisk and vigorous: and if their imaginations were charmed with sweet and melodious airs, and care and thought of business drowned in a glass of rosy wine, that their spirits may be raised to the highest pitch of ardour and joy, it would not be amiss; for any thing of sadness, trouble, and sorrow, are enemies to the delights of Venus. And if, at any such times of coition there should be conception, it would have a malevolent effect upon the child. But though generous restoratives may be used for invigorating nature, yet all excess is to be carefully avoided, for it will allay the briskness of the spirits, and render them dull and languid, and also hinder digestion, and so must needs be an enemy to copulation: for it is food moderately taken and well digested, that creates good spirits, and enables a man with vigour and activity to perform the dictates of nature. It is also highly necessary that in their mutual embraces they meet each other with an equal ardour, for if the spirits flag on either part, they will fall short of what nature requires, and the woman must either miss of conception, or else the children prove weak in their bodies, or defective in their understanding: and therefore I do advise them, before they begin their conjugal embraces, to invigorate their mutual desires, and make their flames burn with a fierce ardour by those endearing ways that love can better teach than I can write.

And when they have done what nature requires, a man must have a care he does not part too soon from the embraces of his wife, lest some sudden interposing cold should strike into the womb, and occasion a miscariage, and thereby deprive them of their labour.

And when, after some small convenient time, the man hath withdrawn himself, let the woman gently betake herself to rest with all imaginable serenity and composure of mind, free from all anxious and disturbing thoughts, or any other kind of perturbation whatsoever. And let her, as much as she can, forbear turning herself from that side on which she first reposed. And by all means let her avoid coughing and sneezing, which, by its violent concussion on the body is a great enemy to conception, if it happen soon after the act of coition.

A PRIVATE LOOKING-GLASS

FOR THE

FEMALE SEX.

PART SECOND.

TREATING OF SEVERAL MALADIES INCIDENT TO THE WOMB, WITH PROPER REMEDIE FOR THE CURE OF EACH.

CHAPTER I.

Of the womb in general.

ALTHOUGH in the first part I have spoken something of the womb, yet being in the second part to treat more particularly thereof, and of the various distempers and maladies it is subjected to, I shall not think it tautology to give you, by way of instruction, a general description both of its situation and extent, but rather think it can by no means be omitted, especially since in it I am to speak of the quality of the menstruous blood.

First, touching the womb. By the Grecians it is called metra, the mother; adelphos, says Priscian because it makes us all brothers.

It is placed in the hypogastrium, or lower part of the body, in the cavity called pelvis, having the strait gut on one side, to keep it from the other side of the backbone, and the bladder on the other side to defend it from blows. The form or figure of it is like a virile-member, only thus described—the manhood is outward, and womanhood inward.

It is divided into the neck and the body. The neck consists of a hard fleshy substance, much like cartilage, to the end whereof there is a membrane transversely placed, called hymen, or engion. Near to the neck there is a prominent pinnacle, which is called by Mountinus, the door of the womb, because it preserves the matrix from cold and dust; by the Grecians it is called clytoris: by the Latins, præputium muliebre, because the Jewish women did abuse those parts to their own mutual lusts, as Paul speaks, Rom. i. 26.

The body of the womb is that wherein the child is conceived; and this is not altogether round, but dilates itself into two angles, the outward part of it nervous and full of sinews, which are the cause of its motion, but inwardly it is fleshy. In the cavity of the womb there are two cells or receptacles for human seed, divided by a line running through the midst of it. In the right side of the cavity, by the reason of the heat of the liver, males are conceived; in the left side, by the coldness of the spleen, females are begotten. Most of our moderns hold the above as an infallible truth; yet Hippocrates holds it but in general: "For in whom (saith he) the spermatic vessels on the right side come from the reins, and the spermatic vessels on the left side from the hollow vein, in them males are conceived in the left side, and females in the right." Well, therefore, may I conclude with the saying of Empedocles. "Such sometimes is the power of the seed, that the male may be conceived in the left side, as well as in the right." In the bottom of the cavity, there are little holes called the cotiledones, which are the ends of certain veins and arteries, serving in breeding women to convey substance to the child, which is received by the umbilical veins; and others to carry their courses into the matrix.

Now, touching the menstruals, they are defined to be a monthly flux of excrementitious and unprofitable blood, which is to be understood of the superplus or redundance of it. For it is an excrement in quality, its quantity being pure and incorrupt, like unto the blood in the veins.

And that the menstruous blood is pure and subtle of itself, all in one quality with that in the veins, is proved two ways: first, from the final cause of the blood, which is the propagation and conversation of mankind, that man might be conceived; and being begotton, he might be comforted and preserved both in the womb and out of the womb. And all will grant it for a truth, that a child, when in the matrix, is nourished with the blood. And it is true, that being out of the womb, it is still nourished with the same; for the milk is nothing but the menstruous blood made white in the breast. Secondly, it is proved to be true, from the generation of it, it being the superfluity of the last aliment of the fleshy parts.

The natural end of man and woman's being is to propagate:

and this injunction was imposed upon them by God at their first creation, and again after the deluge. Now, in the act of conception, there must be an agent and patient; for if they be both every way of one constitution, they cannot propagate: man therefore is hot and dry, woman cold and moist; he is the agent, she the patient or weaker vessel, that she should be subject to the office of the man. It is necessary the woman should be of a cold constitution: because in her is required a redundancy of nature for the infant depending on her; for otherwise, if there were not a superplus of nourishment for the child, more than is convenient for the mother, then would the infant detract and weaken the principal parts of the mother, and like unto the viper, the generation of the infant would be the destruction of the parent.

The monthly purgations continue from the 15th year to the 46th or 50th; yet often there happens a suppression which is either natural or morbifical; they are naturally suppressed in breeding women, and such as give suck. The morbifical suppression falls now into our method to be spoken of.

CHAPTER II.

Of the Retention of the Courses.

The suppression of the terms, is an interception of that accustomed evacuation of blood which every month should come from the matrix, proceeding from the instrument or matter vitiated. The part affected is the womb, and that of itself or by consent.

CAUSE. The cause of this suppression is either external or internal. The external cause may be heat, or dryness of the air, immoderate watching, great labour, vehement motion, &c. whereby the matter is so consumed and the body so exhausted, that there is not a surplus remaining to be expelled, as is recorded of the Amazons, who, being active and always in motion, had their fluxions very little or not at all. Or it may be caused by cold, which is most frequent, making the blood vicious and gross, condensing and binding up the passages that it cannot flow forth.

The internal cause is either instrumental or material, in the womb or in the blood.

In the womb it may be divers ways; by imposthumes, humours, ulcers, by the narrowness of the veins and passages, or by the omentum, in fat bodies, pressing the neck of the matrix: but then they must have hernia, zirthilis, for in mankind the kell reacheth not so low; by overmuch cold or heat, the one vitiating the action, the other consuming the matter; by an evil composition of the uterine parts, by the neck of the womb being turned aside, and sometimes, though rarely, by a membrane or excrescence of the flesh growing about the mouth or neck of the womb. The blood may be in fault two ways, in quantity or quality; in quantity, when it is so consumed that there is not a superplus left, as in viragoes, or virile women, who, through their heat and strength of nature, digest and consume all in their last nourishment, as Hippocrates writes of Prethusa, who being exalted by her husband Pathea, her terms were suppressed, her voice changed, and had a beard, with the countenance of a man. But these I judge rather to be Tynopagi, or woman eaters, than women breeders, because they consume one of the principles of generation, which gives a being to the world, viz. the menstruous blood. The blood likewise may be consumed, and consequently the terms staid, by bleeding at the nose, by a flux of the hemorrhoids, by a dysentery commonly called the bloody flux, by many other evacuations, and by continual and chronical diseases. Secondly, the matter may be vicious in quality; and suppose it to be sanguinous, phlegmatical, bilious, or melancholic; every one of these, if they offend in grossness, will cause an obstruction in the veins.

Signs. Signs manifesting the disease, are pains in the head, neck, back, and loins; weariness of the whole body, but especially of the hips and legs, by reason of a confinity which the matrix have with these parts; trembling of the heart. Particular signs are these: If the suppression proceed from cold, she is heavy, sluggish, of a pale colour, and has a slow pulse: Venus's combats are neglected, the urine cruddles, the blood becomes waterish and much in quantity, and the excrements of the guts usually are retained. If of heat; the signs are contrary to those now recited. If the retention be natural, and come of conception, this may be known by drinking of hydromel, that is, water and honey, after supper, going to bed, by the effect which it worketh; for if, after the taking of it, she feels a beating pain upon the navel, and the lower part of the belly, it is a sign she hath conceived, and that the suppression is natural; if not, then it is vicious, and ought medicinally to be taken away.

Prognostics. With the evil quality of the womb, the whole body stands charged, but especially the heart, the liver, and the brain; and betwixt the womb and these three principal parts there is a singular concert: First, the womb communicates to the heart by the mediation of those arteries which come from the aorta. Hence, the terms being suppressed, will ensue faintings, swoonings, intermission of pulse, cessation of breath. Secondly, it communicates to the liver by the veins derived from the hollow vein. Hence will follow obstructions, cahexies, jaundice, dropsies, hardness of spleen. Thirdly, it communicates to the brain by the nerves and membrane of the back; hence will arise epilepsies, frenzies, melancholy, passion, pain in the afterparts of the head, fearfulness, and inability of speaking. Well, therefore, may I conclude with Hippocrates, if the months be suppressed many dangerous diseases will follow.

CURE. In the cure of this, and of all the other following effects, I will observe the order. The cure shall be taken from chirurgical, pharmaceutical and diuretical means.—This suppression is a plethoric effect, and must be taken away by evacuation, and therefore we will first begin with phlebotomy. In the midst of the menstrual period open the liver vein; and for the reservation of the humour, two days before the evacuation, open the saphena in both feet: if the repletion be not great, apply cupping glasses to the legs and thighs, although there should be no hopes to remove the suppression. As in some the cotiledones are so closed up, that nothing but copulation will open them: yet it will be convenient, as much as may be, to ease nature of her burden, by opening the hemorrhoid veins with a leech. After phlebotomy, let the humours be prepared and made flexible with syrup of stychas calamint, betony, hyssop, mugwort, horehound, fumitary, maiden hair. Bathe with camomile, penny royal, savia, bay leaves, juniper berries. rue, marjoram, feverfew. Take of the leaves of nep, maiden hair, succory, and betony, of each a handful. make a decoction; take thereof three ounces Syrup of maiden hair, mugwort, and succory: mix of each half an ounce After she comes out of the bath, let her drink it off. Purge with pill de agaric: fleybang, corb, feriæ. Galen, in this case, commends pilulæ de caberica, coloquintida; for, as they are proper to purge the humour offending, so also they do open the passage of the womb, and strengthen the faculty by their aromatical quality.

If the stomach be overcharged, let her take a vomit, yet such an one as may work both ways, lest working only upward; it should too much turn back the humour. Take trochisks of agaric two drams, infuse them in two ounces of oxymel, in which dissolve of the electuary diasarum one scruple and a half, bendic. laxit. half an ounce. Take this after the manner of a purge.

After the humour hath been purged, proceed to more proper and forcible remedies. Take of trochisk of myrrh one dram and a half; parsley seed, castor rinds, or cassia, of each one scruple, and of the extract of mugwort one scruple and a half: of musk ten grains, with the juice of smallage: make twelve pills; take six every morning, or after supper going to bed. Take of cinnamon half an ounce, smirutium, or rogos, valeria aristolochia, of each two drams; roots of astrumone, dram saffron, of each two scruples; spec. diembia, two drams; trochisk of myrrh, four scruples; tartari vitriolari, two scruples; make half into a powder with mugwort water and sugar a sufficient quantity; make lozenges; take one dram of them every morning, or mingle one dram of the powder with one dram of sugar, and take it in white wine. Take of prepared steel, spec. hair, of each two drams; borax, spec. of myrrh, of each one scruple, with the juice of savine; make it up into eighty eight lozenges, and take three every other day before dinner. Take of castor one scruple, wild carrot seed half a dram, with syrup of mugwort, and make four pills, take them in a morning fasting, and so for three days together, before the wonted time of the purgation. Take of agaric, aristolochia, juice of horehound, of each five drams; rhubarb, spikenard, anniseed, gaidanum, assafœtida, mallow root, gentian, of the three peppers, lacoac, of each six drams; with honey make an electuary, take of it three drams for a dose. In phlegmatic bodies nothing can be better given than the decoction of the wood of guaicum, with a little disclaim, taken in the morning fasting, and so for twelve days together, without provoking of sweat.

Administer to the lower parts by suffumigations, pessaries, unctions, injections: make suffumigations of cinnamon, nutmeg, cloves, nay berries, mugwort, galbanum, molanthium, amber, &c. Make pessaries of figs, and the leaves of mercury bruised, and rolled up with lint. If you desire a stronger, make one of myrrh, adulium, apopanax, ammoniacum, galbanum, sagepanum, mithridate, agaric, coloquintida, &c. Make injections of the decoction of origane, mugwort, mercury, betony, and eggs; inject it into the womb by an instrument fit for that purpose. Take of oil of almonds, lilies, capers, camomile, of each half an ounce; laudani, oil of myrrh, of each two drams; with wax make an unguent, with which let the place be anointed; make infusions of fenugreek, camomile, melilot, dill, marjoram, pennyroyal, feverfew, juniper berries, and calamint; but if the suppression comes by a defect of matter, then ought not the courses to be provoked until the spirits be animated, and the blood again increased: or if by proper effects of the womb as dropsies, inflamations, &c. then must particular care be used; the which I will not insist upon here, but speak of them as they lie in order.

If the retention comes from repletion or fulness, if the air be hot and dry, use moderate exercise before meals, and your meat and drink attenuating; use with your meat garden savory, thyme, origane, and eyche peason: if of emptiness, or defect of matter, if the air be moist and moderately hot, shun exercise and watching; let your meat be nourishing and of light digestion, as raw eggs, lamb, chickens, almonds, milk, and the like.

CHAPTER III.

Of the Overflowing of the Courses.

The learned say, that by comparing contraries, truth is made manifest; having therefore spoken of the suppression of terms, order requires now that I should insist on the overflowing of them an effect no less dangerous than the former; and this immoderate flux of the mouth is defined to be a sanguinous excrement, proceeding from the womb, exceeding both in quantity and time. First, it is said to be sanguinous, the matter of the flux being only blood, wherein it differs from that which is commonly called the false courses, or the whites, of which I shall speak hereafter. Secondly, it is said to proceed from the womb: for there are two ways from which the blood flows forth; the one is by the internal views of the body of the womb; and this is properly called the monthly flux; the other is by those veins which are terminated in the neck of the matrix; and this is called by Aetius, the hemorrhoids of the womb. Lastly, it is said to exceed both in quantity and time. In quantity, saith Hippocrates, when they flow about eighteen ounces; in time, when they flow above three days; but we take this for a certain character of their inordinate flowing, when the faculties of the body are thereby weakened. In bodies abounding in gross humours, this immoderate flux sometimes unburdens nature of her load, and aught not to be staid without the counsel of a physician.

Cause. The cause of this affair is internal or external. The internal cause is threefold; in the matter, instrument, or faculty. The matter, which is the blood, may be vicious two ways; first, by the heat of constitution, climate, or season, heating the blood, whereby the passages are dilated, and the faculty weakened, that it cannot retain the blood. Secondly, by falls, blows, violent motion, breaking of the veins,

&c. The external cause may be calidity of the air, lifting, carrying of heavy burdens, unnatural child-birth, &c.

SIGNS. In this inordinate flux the appetite is decayed, the conception is depraved, and all the actions weakened; the feet are swelled, the colour of the face is changed, and a general feebleness possesseth the whole body. If the flux comes by the breaking of a vein, the body is sometimes cold, the blood flows forth in heaps, and that suddenly, with great pains. If it comes through heat, the orifice of the vein being diluted, then there is little or no pain, yet the blood flows faster than it doth in an erosion, and not so fast as it doth in a rupture. If by erosion, or sharpness of blood, she feels a great heat scalding the passage; it differs from the other two, in that it flows not so suddenly, nor so copiously as they do. If by weakness of the womb, she abhorreth the use of Venus. Lastly, if it proceed from an evil quality of the blood, drop some of it on a cloth, and when it is dry, you may judge of the quality by the colour. If it be choleric, it will be yellow; if melancholy, black; if phlegmatic, waterish and whitish.

PROGNOSTICS. If with the flux be joined a convulsion, it is dangerous, because it intimates the more noble parts are vitiated: and a convulsion caused by emptiness is deadly. If it continues long, it will be cured with great difficulty: for it was one of the miracles which our Saviour, Christ, wrought, to cure this disease, when it had continued twelve years.

To conclude, if the flux be inordinate, many diseases will ensue, and without remedy, the blood, together with the native heat, being consumed, either cachetical, hydropical, or paralytical diseases will follow.

CURE. The cure consisteth in three particulars. First, in repelling and carrying away the blood: Secondly, in correcting and taking away the fluxibility of the matter: Thirdly, in incorporating the veins and faculties. For the first, to cause a regression of the blood, open a vein in the arm, and draw out so much blood as the strength of the patient will permit; and that not altogether, but at several times, for thereby the spirits are less weakened, and the refraction so much the greater.

Apply cupping-glasses to the breasts, and also the liver, that the reversion may be in the fountain.

To correct the fluxibility of the matter, cathartical means, moderated with the astrictories, may be used.

If it be caused by erosion, or sharpness of blood, consider whether the erosion be by salt phlegm, or adust choler. If by salt phlegm, prepare with syrup of violets, wormwood, roses, citron-pill, succory, &c. Then make this purgation following: mirobolans, chebol, half an ounce trochisks of agaric, one dram; with plantain-water, make a decoction; add thereto fir, roast, and lax; three ounces, and make a potion.

If by adust choler, prepare the body with syrup of roses, myrtles, sorrel, and purslain, mixed with water of plantain, knot-grass, and endive. Then purge with this potion; take rind of mirobolans and rhubarb of each one dram, cinnamon fifteen grains; infuse them one night in endive water; add to the straining, pulp of tamarind, cassia, of each half an ounce, syrup of roses an ounce; make a potion. If the blood be waterish or uncocted, as it is in hydropical bodies, and flows forth by reason of the tenacity or thinness, to draw off the water, it will be profitable to purge with agaric, elaterium, coloquintida; sweating is proper in this case, for thereby the matter offending is taken away, and the motion of the blood carried to the outward parts. To procure sweat, use cardus-water, with mithridate, or the decoction of guaiacum and sarsaparilla. The gum of guaiacum: also doth greatly provoke sweat: pills of sarsaparilla, taken every night going to bed, are worthily recommended. If the blood flows forth through the opening or breaking of a vein, without any evil quality of itself, then ought only corroboratives to be applied; which is the last thing to be done in this inordinate flux.

Take of bole ammoniac one scruple, London treacle one dram, old conserve of roses half an ounce, with syrup of myrtle make an electuary; or, if the flux hath continued long, take of mastic two drams, olibani troch de caraba, of each one dram; balustium one scruple: make a powder: with syrup of quinces make it into pills: take one always before meals. Take lapidis, hæmatia, triti, of each two scruples; spederdum, alantalia, one ounce; treeh decarabede, scorria, ferri, coral, frankincense, of each one scruple; fine bole one scruple; beat these to fine powder, and with sugar and plaintain-water make lozenges. Asses' dung is approved of, whether token inwardly with syrup of quinces, or outwardly with steeled-water. Galen, by conveying the juice of it through a metrenchita in the womb four days together, cured this immoderate flux, which no ways else could be restrained. Going to bed, let her take one scruple and a half of pilon in water; make a suffumigation for the matrix of mastic, frankincense, burnt frogs, not forgetting the hoof of a mule. Take the juice of knot-grass, comfrey, and quinces, of each one ounce, camphire one dram, dip silk or cotton therein, and apply it to the place. Take of oil of mastic, myrtles, quinces, of each half an ounce; fine bole, troch, decarda, of each one dram; sanguis draconis a sufficient quantity; make an unguent, and apply it before and behind. Take of plantain, shepherd's purse, red rose leaves, of each one ounce and a half; dried mint one ounce; bean-meal three ounces: boil all these in plantain-water, and make of it two plaisters, apply one before and behind. If the blood flow from those veins which are terminated in the neck of the matrix, then it is not called the overflowing of the terms, but the hemorrhoids of the womb; yet the same cure will serve both, only the instrumental cure will a little differ: for, in the uterine hermorrhoids, the ends of the veins hang over like little teats or brushes, which must be taken away by incision: and then the veins closed up with aloes. fine bole, burnt allum, trorch de terrs fiall; myrrh, mastic, with the juice of comfrey and knot-grass, laid plaisterways thereunto.

The air must be cold and dry. All motion of the body must be forbidden. Let her meat be pleasant. patridge, mountain birds, coneys, calf feet. &c. And let her beer be mixed with juice of pomegranates and quinces.

CHAPTER IV.
Of the Weeping of the Womb.

THE weeping of the womb is a flux of blood, unnatural, coming from thence by drops, after the manner of tears, causing violent pains in the same, keeping neither period nor time. By some it is referred unto the immoderate evacuation of the courses, yet they are distinguished in the quantity and manner of overflowing. in that they flow copiously and free; this is continual. though by little and little, and that with great pain and difficulty: wherefore it is likened unto the stranguary.

The cause is in the faculty, instrument, or matter: in the faculty, by being enfeebled that it cannot expel the blood; and the blood resting there. make that part of the womb grow hard. and stretcheth the vessels; from whence proceed the pains of the womb. In the instrument, by the narrowness of the passages. Lastly, it may be the matter of the blood, which may offend in too great a quantity or in an evil quality, it being so gross and thick that it cannot flow forth as it ought to do, but by drops. The signs will best appear by the relation of the patient: hereupon will issue pains in the head, stomach, and back, with inflamations, suffocations, and excoriations of the matrix. If the strength of the patient will permit, first open a vein in the arm, rub the upper parts, and let her arm be corded, that the force of the blood may be carried backward: then apply such things as may laxate and molify the strengthening of the womb, and assuage the sharpness of the blood, as cataplasms made of bran, linseed, fenugreek, melilot, mallows, mercury, and artiplex. If the blood be vicious and gross, add thereto mugwort, calamint, dictam, and betony; and let her take of Venice treacle the quantity of a nutmeg and the syrup of mugwort every morning; make an injection of the decoction of mallows, mercury, linseed, groundsel, mugwort, fenugreek, with oil of sweet almonds.

Sometimes it is caused by the wind, and then phlebotomy is to be omitted, and in the stead thereof, take syrup of feverfew one ounce: honey, roses, syrup of roses, syrup of flachus, of each half an ounce: water of calamint, mugwort, betony, and hyssop, of each one ounce, make a julep. If the pain continues, take this purgation: take of spec. and hieræ one dram, diacatholicon half an ounce; syrup of roses and laxative one ounce; with the decoction of mugwort and the four cordial flowers make a potion. If it comes through the weakness of the faculty, let them be corroborated. If through the grossness and sharpness of the blood, let the quality of it be altered, as I have shown in the foregoing chapter. Lastly, if the excrement of the guts be retained, provoke them by a clyster of the decoction of camomile, betony, feverfew, mallows, linseed, juniper berries, cummin seed, anniseed, melilot, adding thereto of diacatholicon half an ounce; hiera picra, two drams; honey and oil of each one ounce; salt-nitre a dram and a half. The patient must abstain from salt, sharp and windy meats.

CHAPTER V.

Of the False Corses, or Whites.

FROM the womb proceed not only menstruous blood, but, accidentally, many other excrements, which by the ancients are comprehended under the title of rebus gunakois; which is a distillation of a variety of corrupt humour through the womb, flowing from the whole body, or a part of the same, keeping neither courses nor colour, but varying in both.

CAUSE. The cause is either promiscuously in the whole body, by a cocochymia, or weakness of the same, or in some of the parts, as in the liver, which, by the inability of the sanguificative faculty, causeth a generation of corrupt blood, and then the matter is reddish; sometimes the gall being sluggish in its office, not drawing away those choleric superfluities engendered in the liver, the matter is yellowish; sometimes in the spleen, not deficiating and cleansing the blood of the dregs and excrementitious parts; and then the matter flowing forth is blackish. It may also come from the catarrh in the head, or from any other putrified or corrupted member; but if the matter of the flux be white, the cause is either in the stomach or reigns: in the stomach by a phlegmatical and crude matter there contracted and vitiated, through grief, melancholy and other distempers; for, otherwise, if the matter were only pituitous, crude phlegm, and no ways corrupt, being taken into the liver, it might be converted into blood; for phlegm in the ventricle is called nourishment half digested: but being corrupt, though sent into the liver, yet it cannot be turned into nutriment: for the second decoction cannot correct that which the first hath corrupted; and therefore the liver sends it to the womb, which can neither digest nor repel it, and so it is voided out with the same colour it had in the ventricle. The cause also may be in the reins being overheated, whereby the spermatical matter, by reason of its thinness, flows forth. The external causes may be moistness of the air, eating of corrupt meats, anger, grief, slothfulness, immoderate sleeping, costiveness in the body.

The signs are, extenuation of the body, shortness and stinking of the breath, loathing of meat, pain in the head, swellings of the eyes and feet, and melancholy; humidity flows from the womb of divers colours, as red, black, green, yellow, and white. It differs from the flowing and overflowing of the courses, in that it keeps no certain period, and is of many colours, all of which do generate from blood.

Prognostic. If the flux be phlegmatical, it will continue long and be difficult to cure, yet if vomiting or diarrhœa happeneth, it diverts the humour and cures the disease. If it be choleric, it is not so permanent, yet more perilous, for it will cause a cliff in the neck of the womb, and sometimes make an excoriation of the matrix; if melancholic, it must be dangerous and contumacious. Yet the flux of the hemorrhoids administer cure.

If the matter flowing forth be reddish, open a vein in the arm: if not, apply ligatures to the arms and shoulders. Galen glories of himself, how he cured the wife of Brutus, labouring of this disease, by rubbing the upper part with crude honey.

If it be caused by a distillation from the brain, take syrup of betony, stochas, and marjoram: purge with pillcoen, fine quibus de agrico: make nasalia of the juice of sage, hyssop, betony, nigella, with one drop of oil of elect. dianth, aromat.

rosat, diambre, diamosei dulcis, of each one dram, nutmeg half a dram: with sugar and betony water make lozenges, to be taken every morning and evening; Auri Alexandria, half a dram at night going to bed. If these things help not, use the suffumigation and plaister, as they are prescribed.

If it proceed from crudities in the stomach, or from a cold distempered liver, take every morning of the decoction of lignum sanctum: purge with pill de agrico, de hermodact, de hiera, diacolinthio, fætid. agrigatio: take elect aromat. roses two drams; citron peel dried, nutmeg, long pepper, of each one scruple; diaglanga one dram: fantali, alb. lign. aloes, of each half a scruple; sugar six ounces, with mint water; and make lozenges of it; take of them before meals. If, with the frigidity of the liver, there be joined a repletion of the stomach, purging by vomit is commendable; for which three drams of the electuary diasatu. Galen allows of diuretical means, as absum petrofolman.

If the matter of the flux be choleric, prepare the humour with syrup of roses, violets, endive, succory; purge with mirobolans, manna, rhubarb, cassia. Take of rhubarb two drams, anniseed one dram, cinnamon a scruple and a half; infuse them in six ounces of prune-broth, add of the straining of manna one ounce, and take in the morning according to art. Take specierum, diatonlantoe, diacorant, prig, diarthod, abbaris, dyacydomes, of each one dram. sugar four ounces, with plantain water; make lozenges. If the clyster of the gall be sluggish, and do not stir up the faculty of the gut, give hot clysters of the decoction of the four mollifying herbs with honey of roses and aloes.

If the flux be melancholous, prepare with syrup of maidenhair, epithymium, polipoly, borrage, buglos, fumitary, hartstongue, and syrupus bisantius, which must be made without vinegar, otherwise it will rather animate the disease than nature: for melancholy by the use of vinegar is increased, and both by Hippocrates, Silvius, and Avenzoar, it is disallowed of as an enemy to the womb, and therefore not to be used inwardly in all uterine diseases. Purgers of melancholy are pilulæ sumariœ, pilulæ lud de lapina, lazuli diosena, and confectio hamec. Take of stamped prunes two ounces; sen. one dram; epithimium, polibody, fumitary, of each a dram and a half; sour dates, one ounce; with endive water, make a decoction; take of it four ounces, add unto it confections, hamesech three drams, manna three drams. Or take pil. indie, pil. fœtid. agarici, trochisati, of each one scruple; pills of rhubarb one scruple: lapidis lazuli six grains; with syrup of epithimium make pills, and take them once every week. Take elect. lætificants, galen three drams;

diamargarita, calimlone, diamosci, dulcis, conservei of borage, violets, bugloss, of each a dram; citron-peel candied one dram; sugar seven ounces; with rose water make lozenges.

Lastly, Let the womb be cleansed from the corrupt matter, and then corroborated. For the purifying thereof, make injections of the decoction of betony, feverfew, spikenard, bistort, mercury, and sage, adding thereto sugar, oil of sweet almonds, of each two ounces; pessaries also may be made of silk or cotton, mollified in the juice of the aforenamed herbs.

To corroborate the womb, you must thus prepare trochisks; take of mugwort, feverfew, myrrh, amber, mace, nutmeg, storax, lign aloes, red roses, of each one ounce: with the mucilage, tragacanth, make trochisks; cast some of them into coals, and smoke the womb therewith, and make fomentations for the womb with red wine, in which hath been decocted mastic, fine bole, malustia, and red roots; anoint the matrix with oil of quinces and myrtles, and apply thereto emplastrum, pro matrice; and let her take diamosdum, dulce, aract, and celematicum, every morning.

A dry diet is commended to be the best, because in this effect the body most commonly abounds with phlegmatical and crude humours. For this cause Hippocrates counsels the patient to go to bed supperless. Let her meat be partridge, pheasant, and mountain birds, rather roasted than boiled. Immoderate sleep is forbidden, moderate exercise is commended.

CHAPTER II.

Of the Suffocation of the Mother.

This effect, which, if simply considered, is nothing but the cause of an effect, is called in English, "The suffocation of the mother;" not because the womb is strangled, but for that it causeth the womb to be choked. It is a retraction of the womb towards the midriff and the stomach, which so presseth and crusheth up the same, that the instrumental cause of respiration, the midriff, is suffocated, and consenting with the brain, causes the animating faculty, the efficient cause of respiration, also to be intercepted, while the body being refrigerated, and the action depraved, she falls to the ground as one dead.

In those hysterical passions some continue longer, some shorter. Rabbi Moses writes of some who lay in the paroxysm of the fit for two days. Rufus makes mention of one who continued in the same passion three days and three nights; and at the three days end she revived That we may learn by other men's harms to beware, I will tell you an example: Paroetus writeth of a woman in Spain, who suddenly fell into an uterine suffocation, and appeared to men's judgment as dead; her friends wondering at this her sudden change, for their better satisfaction sent for a surgeon to have her dissected, who, beginning to make an incision, the woman began to move, and with great clamour returned to herself again, to the horror and admiration of the spectators.

To the end that you may distinguish the living from the dead, the ancients prescribe three experiments: the first is, to lay a light feather to the mouth, and by its motion you may judge whether the patient be living or dead: the second is, to place a glass of water on the breast, and if you perceive it to move, it betokeneth life: the third is, to hold a pure looking glass to the mouth and nose; and if the glass appears thick, with a little dew upon it, it betokeneth life: and these three experiments are good, yet with this caution, that you ought not to depend upon them too much: for though the feather and the water do not move, and the glass continue pure and clear, yet it is not a necessary consequence that she is destitute of life. For the motion of the lungs, by which the respiration is made, may be taken away that she cannot breathe, yet the internal transpiration of the heat may remain; which is not manifest by the motion of the breast or lungs, but lies occult in the heart and inward arteries: examples whereof we have in the fly and swallow, who, in cold winters, to occular aspect, seem dead, inanimate, and breathe not at all: yet they live by the transpiration of that heat which is reserved in the heart and inward arteries: therefore, when the summer approacheth, the internal heat being revocated to the outward parts, they are then again revived out of their sleepy extasy.

Those women, therefore, who seem to die suddenly, and upon no evident cause, let them not be committed unto the earth until the end of three days, lest the living be buried for the dead.

Cure. The part effected is the womb, of which there is a twofold motion—natural and symptomatical. The natural motion is, when the womb attracteth the human seed, or excludeth the infant or secundine. The symptomatical motion, of which we are to speak, is a convulsive drawing up of the womb.

The cause usually is in the retention of the seed, or the suppression of the menses, causing a repletion of the corrupt humours in the womb, from whence proceeds a flatuous refrigeration, causing a convulsion of the ligaments of the womb. And as it may come from humidity or repletion, being a convulsion, it may be caused by emptiness or dryness. And lastly, by abortion, or difficult child-birth.

SIGNS. At the approaching of the suffocation, there is a paleness of the face, weakness of the legs, shortness of breath, frigidity of the whole body, with a working into the throat, and then she falls down as one void of both sense and motion; the mouth of the womb is closed up, and being touched with the finger, feels hard. The paroxysm of the fit being once past, she openeth her eyes, and feeling her stomach oppressed, she offers to vomit. And lest any one should be deceived in taking one disease for another, I will shew how it may be distinguished from those diseases which have the nearest affinity to it.

It differs from the apoplexy, by reason it comes without shrieking out; also in the hysterical passion the sense of feeling is not altogether destroyed and lost, as it is in the apoplectic disease; and it differs from the epilepsies in that the eyes are not wrested, neither doth any spungy froth come from the mouth; and that convulsive motion, which sometimes, and that often, is joined to suffocations, is not universal, as it is in the epilepsies, only this or that matter is convulsed, and that without any vehement agitation. In the syncope, both respiration and pulse are taken away, the countenance waxeth pale, and she swoons away suddenly; but in the hysterical passion, commonly, there is both respiration and pulse, though it cannot be well perceived; her face looks red, and she hath a forewarning of her fit. Yet it is not denied but that syncope may be joined with this suffocation. Lastly, it is distinguished from the lethargy by the pulse, which, in the one is great, and in the other little.

PROGNOSTIC. If the disease hath its being from the corruption of the seed, it foretels more danger than if it proceed from the suppression of the courses, because the seed it concocted, and of a purer quality than the menstruous blood; and the more pure being corrupted, becomes the more foul and filthy, as appears in eggs, the purest nourishment, which, vitiated, yield the noisomest savour. If it be accompanied with a syncope, it shows nature is but weak, and that the spirits are almost exhausted; but if sneezing follows, it shows the heat, which was almost extinct, doth now begin to return, and that nature will subdue the disease.

CURE. In the cure of this effect, two things must be observed: first, that during the time of the paroxysm, nature be provoked to expel those malignant vapours which blind up the senses, that she may be recalled out of that sleepy extasy. Secondly, that in the intermission of the fit, proper medicines may be applied to take away the cause.

To stir up nature, fasten cupping-glasses to the hips and navel, apply ligatures unto the thigh, rub the extreme parts with salt, vinegar, and mustard: cause loud clamours and thundering in the ears. Apply to the nose assafœtida, castor, and sagapaneux, steeped in vinegar: provoke her to sneeze by blowing up into her nostrils the powder of castor, white pepper, Spanish pelitory, and hellebore: hold under her nose partridge feathers, hair, and burnt leather, or any other thing having a strong stinking smell; for evil odours being disagreeable to nature, the animal spirits do so contest and strive against them, that the natural heat is thereby restored. The brain is sometimes so oppressed, that there is a necessity for burning the outward skin of the head with hot oil, or with a hot iron. Sharp clysters and suppositories are available. Take of sage, calamint, horehound, feverfew, marjoram, betony, hyssop, of each one handful: anniseed half an ounce; coloquintida, white hellebore, sal gem, of each two drams; boil these in two pounds of water to the half: add the straining oil of castor two ounces, hiera picra two drams, and make a clyster of it; or, take honey boiled two ounces, cuphorb half a scruple, coloquint four grains, with hellebore two grains, salt one dram; make a suppository. Hippocrates writeth of a hysterical woman, who could not be freed from the paroxysm but by pouring cold water upon her; yet this cure is singular, and ought to be administered only in heat of summer, when the sun is in the tropic of Cancer.

If it be caused by the retention and corruption of the seed, at the instant of the paroxysm, let the midwife take oil of lilies, marjoram, and bays, dissolving in the same two grains of civet, and as much musk: let her dip her finger therein, and put it up into the neck of the womb tickling and rubbing the same.

The fit being over, proceed to the curing of the cause. If it arise from the suppression of the menses, look to the cure in chap. xi. If from the retention of the seed, a good husband will administer a cure: but those who cannot honestly purchase that cure, must use such things as will dry up and diminish the seed, as diacimina, diacalaminthes, &c. Amongst potions, the seed of agnus castus is well esteemed of, whether taken inwardly, applied outwardly, or received as suffumigation; it was held in great honour amongst the Athenians, for by it they did remain as pure vessels and preserved their chastity, by only strewing it on the bed whereon they lay, and hence the name of agnus castus given it, as denoting its effects. Make an issue on the inside of each leg, a handbreadth below the knee. Make trochisks of agaric, two scruples, wild carrot seed, lign. aloes, of each half a scruple; washed turpentine, three drams; with conserve of anthos make a bolus. Castor is of excellent use in this case, eight drams of it taken in white wine; or you may make pills of it with mithridate, and take them going to bed. Take of white briony root, dried and cut after the manner of carrots, one ounce, put in a draught of wine, placing it by the fire, and when it is warm, drink it. Take myrrh, castor and assafœtida, of each one scruple; saffron and rue-seed, of each four grains; make eight pills, and take two every night going to bed.

Galen, by his own example, commends unto us agaric pulverized, of which he frequently gave one scruple in white wine. Lay to the navel, at bed time, a head of garlic bruised, fastening it with a swathing-band. Make a girdle of galbanum for the waist, and also a plaister for the belly, placing in one part of it civet and musk, which must be laid upon the navel. Take pulveris, benedict, trochisk of agaric, of each two drams; of mithridate a sufficient quantity; and so make two pessaries, and it will purge the matrix of wind and phlegm; foment the natural part with salid oil, in which hath been boiled rue, feverfew, and camomile. Take of rose leaves a handful, cloves two scruples: quilt them in a little cloth, and boil them in malmsey the eighth part of an hour, and apply them to the mouth of the womb, as hot as may be endured, but let not the smell go to her nose. A dry diet must still be observed. The moderate use of Venus is commended. Let her bread be anniseed biscuit, her flesh meat rather roasted than boiled.

CHAPTER VII.

Of the descending or falling of the Mother

THE falling down of the womb is a relaxation of the ligatures, whereby the matrix is carried backward, and in some hangs out in the bigness of an egg; of this there are two kinds, distinguished by a descending and precipitation. The descending of the womb is, when it sinks down to the entrance of the privities, and appears to the eye either not at all, or very little. The precipitation is, when the womb, like a purse, is turned inside outward, and hangs betwixt the thighs in the bigness of a cupping-glass.

CAUSE. The cause is external or internal; the external cause is difficult child-birth, violent pulling away of the secundine, rashness and inexperience in drawing away the child, violent coughing, sneezing, falls, blows, and carrying heavy burdens. The internal cause in general is overmuch humidity flowing into these parts, hindering the operations of the womb, whereby the ligaments by which the womb is supported are relaxed.

The cause in particular is referred to be in the retention of the seed, or in the suppression of the monthly courses.

SIGNS. The arse-gut and bladder oftentimes are so crushed that the passage of both the excrements are hindered; if the urine flows forth white and thick, and the midriff moistened, the loins are grieved, the privities pained, and the womb sinks down to the private parts, or else comes clean out.

PROGNOSTICS. This grief possessing an old woman, is cured with great difficulty: because it weakens the faculties of the womb, and therefore, though it be reduced into its proper place, yet upon every little illness or indisposition, it is subject to return; and so it also is with the younger sort, if the disease be inveterate. If it be caused by a putrefaction of the nerves, it is incurable.

CURE. The womb being naturally placed between the straight-gut and the bladder, and now fallen down, ought not to be put up again, until the faculty, both of the gut and of the bladder, be stirred up. Nature being unloaded of her burden, let the woman be laid on her back in such sort that her legs may be higher than her head; let her feet be drawn up to her hinder parts, with her knees spread abroad: then molify the swelling with oil of lilies and sweet almonds, or with the decoction of mallows, beets, fenugreek, and linseed; when the inflammation is dissipated let the midwife anoint her hand with oil of mastic, and reduce the womb into its place. The matrix being up, the situation of the patient must be changed, let her legs be put out at length, and laid together: six cupping-glasses to her breasts and navel: boil mugwort, feverfew, red roses, and comfreg in red wine; make suffumigation for the matrix, and move sweet odours to her nose; and at her coming out of the bath, give her of syrup of feverfew one ounce, with a dram of mithridate. Take laudani, mastic, of each three drams, make a plaister of it for the navel; then make pessaries of assafœtida, saffron, comfrey, and mastic, adding thereto a little castor.

The practice of Parius in this case was to make them only of cork, in figure like a little egg, covering them over with wax and mastic, dissolved together, fastening them to a thread, and put into the womb.

The present danger being now taken away, and the matrix seated in its natural abode, the remote cause must be removed. If the body be plethoric, open a vein; prepare with syrup of betony, calamint, hyssop, and feverfew; purge with pil. hierac, agaric, pil. de colcocin. If the stomach be oppressed with crudities, unburden it by vomiting: sudorifical decoctions of lignum sanctum, and sassafras, taken twenty days together, dry up the superfluous moisture, and consequently suppress the cause of the disease.

Let the air be hot and dry, your diet hot and attenuating; abstain from dancing, leaping, squeezing, and from all motion both of body and mind; eat sparingly, drink little, sleep moderately.

CHAPTER VIII.

Of the Inflammation of the Womb.

THE phlegmon, or inflammation of the matrix, is an humour possessing the whole womb, accompanied with unnatural heat, by obstruction, and gathering together of corrupt blood.

CAUSE. The cause of this effect is suppression of the menses, repletion of the whole body, immoderate use of Venus, often handling the genitals, difficult childbirth, vehement agitation of the body, falls, blows; to which also may be added, the use of sharp pessaries, whereby not seldom the womb is inflamed; cupping-glasses also fastened to the pubis and hypogastrium, draw the humours to the womb.

SIGNS. The signs are, anguish, humours, pain in the head and stomach; vomiting, coldness of the knees, convulsions of the neck, doating, trembling of the heart; often there is a straightness of breath, by reason of the heat which is communicated to the midriff, the breasts sympathising with the womb, pained and swelled. Further, if the fore part of the matrix be inflamed, the privities are grieved, the urine is suppressed, or flows forth with difficulty. If the after part, the loins and back suffer, the excrements are retained on the right side, the right hip suffers, the right leg is heavy and slow to motion, insomuch that sometimes she seems to halt; and so if the left side of the womb be inflamed, the left hip is pained, and the left leg is weaker than the right. If the neck of the womb be refreshed, the midwife putting up her finger, shall feel the mouth of it retracted, and closed up with a hardness about it.

PROGNOSTICS. All inflammations of the womb are dangerous, if not deadly; and especially if the total substance of the matrix be inflamed; but they are very perilous if in the neck of the womb. A flue in the belly foretels health, if it be natural; for nature works best by the use of her own instruments.

CURE. In cure, first let the humours flowing to tne womb be repelled; for effecting of which, after the belly has been loosed by cooling clysters, phlebotomy will be needful; open therefore a vein in the arm, if she be not with child; the day after strike the saphena on both feet, fasten ligatures and cupping-glasses to the arm, and rub the upper part. Purge gently with cassia, rhubarb, senna, myrobolans. Take of senna two drams, anniseed one scruple, myrobolans half an ounce, barley-water a sufficient quantity: make a decoction; dissolve it in syrup of succory, with rhubarb two ounces, pulp of cassia half an ounce, oil of anniseed two drops, and make a potion. At the beginning of the disease anoint the privities and reins with oil of roses and quinces: make plaisters of plantain, linseed, barley-meal, melilot, fenugreek, whites of eggs, and, if the pain be vehement, a little opium; foment the genitals with the decoction of poppy heads, purslain, knot-grass, and water-lilies; then make injections of goat's milk, rose-water, clarafied whey, with honey of roses. In the declining of the disease, use incisions of sage, linseed, mugwort, pennyroyal, horehound, and fenugreek; anoint the lower part of the belly with the oil of camomile and violets.

Take lily-roots and mallow-roots, of each four ounces; mercury one handful; mugwort, and feverfew, camomile flowers, and melilot, of each a handful and a half; bruise the herbs and roots, and boil them in a sufficient quantity of milk; then add fresh butter, oil of camomile, and lilies, of each two ounces: bean-meal a sufficient quantity: make two plaisters, the one before, the other behind.

If the tumor cannot be removed, but tends to suppuration, take fenugreek, mallow-roots, decocted figs, linseed, barley-meal, dove's dung, turpentine, of each three drams; deer's suit half a dram, opium half a scruple; with wax make a plaister.

Take of bay leaves, sage, hyssop, camomile, mugwort, and with water make an infusion.

Take wormwood and betony, of each half a handful; white wine and milk, of each half a pound; boil them until one part be confirmed: then take of this decoction four ounces, honey of roses two ounces, and make an injection. Yet beware that the humours are not brought down unto the womb. Take roasted figs and mercury bruised, of each three drams; turpentine and duck's grease, of each three drams: opium, two grains; with wax make a pessary.

The air must be cold; and all the motion of the body, especially of the lower part, is forbidden. Vigilence is commended, for by sleep the humours are carried inward, by which the inflammation is increased; eat sparingly; let your drink be barley water, or clarified whey, and your meat be chickens, and chicken broth, boiled with endive, succory, sorrel, bugloss, and mallows.

CHAPTER IX.

Of the Schirrosity, or Hardness of the Womb.

Of phlegm neglected, or not perfectly cured, is generated a schirrus of the matrix, which is a hard unnatural swelling, insensibly hindering the operations of the womb, and disposing the whole body to slothfulness.

Cause. One cause of this disease may be ascribed to want of judgment in the physician; as many empiricks administering to an inflammation of the womb, do overmuch refrigerate and affrige the humour, that it can neither pass forward nor backward; hence the matter being condensed, degenerates into a lapidious hard substance. Other causes may be suppression of the menstruous retention of the lochi, commonly called the after purgings; eating of corrupt meats, as in the disordinate longing called pica, to which breeding women are so often subject. It may proceed also from obstructions and ulcers in the matrix, or from evil effects in the liver and spleen.

SIGNS. If the bottom of the womb be affected, she feels as it were a heavy burden representing a mole; yet differing, in that the breasts are attenuated, and the whole body waxed less. If the neck of the womb be affected, no outward humours will appear: the mouth of it is retracted, and being touched with the fingers, feels hard, nor can she have the company of a man without great pains and prickings.

PROGNOSTICS. A schirrus confirmed is incurable, and will turn into a cancer, or incurable dropsy; and ending in a cancer, proves deadly, because the native heat in those parts being almost smothered can hardly again be restored.

CURE. Where there is a repletion, phlebotomy is adviseable; wherefore open the medina on both arms, and the saphena on both feet, more especially if the menses be suppressed.

Prepare the humour with syrup of borage, succory, epithyman, and clarified whey: then take of these pills following, according to the strength of the patient:

Take of hiera picra six drams, black helebore, polybody, of each two drams and a half; agaric, lapis lazuli, abluti sa, lindiæ coloquintida, of each one dram and a half; mix them and make pills. The body being purged, proceed to molify the hardness as followeth: anoint the privities and neck of the womb with unguent, decalthea, and agrippa; or take opopanax, bdellium, ammoniac, and myrrh, of each two drams, saffron half a dram; dissolve the gum in oil of lilies and sweet almonds; with wax and turpentine make an unguent; apply below the navel ciacalion, ferellia: make infusions of figs, mugwort, mallows, penny-royal, althea, fennel roots, melilot, fenugreek, boiled in water. Make an injection of calamint, linseed, melilot, fenugreek, and the four mollifying herbs, with oil of dill, camomile, and lilies dissolved in the same. Three draws of the gum bdellium; cast the stone pyrites on the coals, and let her receive the fume into her womb. Foment the secret parts with decoction of the roots and leaves of danewort. Take of gum galbanum, opopanax, of each one dram, juice of danewort, mucilage, fenugreek, of each one dram; calf's marrow an ounce, wax a sufficient quantity: make a pessary, or make a pessary only of lead, dipping it in the aforesaid things, and so put up.

The air must be temperate: gross, vicious, and salt meats are forbidden, as pork, bull's beef, fish, old cheese, &c.

CHAPTER X.

Of the Dropsy of the Womb.

THE uterine dropsy is an unnatural swelling, elevated by the gathering together of wind or phlegm in the cavity, membranes, or substance of the womb, by reason of the debility of the native heat and aliment received, and so it turns into an excrement.

The causes are overmuch cold or moistness of the melt and liver, immoderate drinking, eating of crude meats; all which, causing a repletion, do suffocate the natural heat. It may be caused likewise by the overflowing of the courses, or by any other immoderate evacuation. To these may be added abortions, phlegmons and schirrosities of the womb.

CURE. The signs of this effect are these. The lower parts of the belley, with the genitals, are puffed up, and pained; the feet swell, the natural colour of the face decays, the appetite is depraved, and the heaviness of the whole body concurs. If she turns herself in the bed, from one side to the other, a noise like the flowing of water is heard. Water sometimes comes from the matrix. If the swelling be caused by wind, the belley being hot, it sounds like a drum; the guts rumble, and the wind breaks through the neck of the womb with a murmuring noise; this effect may be distinguished from a true conception many ways, as will appear by the chapter "Of Conception." It is distinguished from the general dropsy, in that the lower parts of the belly are most swelled. Again, in this sanguificative faculty it appears not so hurtful, nor the urine so pale, nor the countenance so soon changed, neither are the superior parts extenuated as in the general dropsy.

PROGNOSTICS. This effect foretells the sad ruin of the natural functions, by that singular consent the womb hath with the liver, and that therefore chachevy, or general dropsy, will follow.

CURE. In the cure of this disease imitate the practice of Hippocrates: first, mitigate the pain with fomentation of melilot, mercury, mallows, linseed, camomile, and althea; then let the womb be prepared with syrup of stœbis, hyssop, calamint, mugwort, of both sorts, with the distilled waters or decoction of elder, marjoram, sage, origan, sperage, pennyroyal, betony: purge with senna, agaric, rhubarb, and claterium. Take specierum, hier, rhubarb, and trochisks of agaric, of each one scruple; with juice of iros make pills.

In diseases which have their rise from moistness, purge with pills. And in these effects which are caused by emptiness or dryness, purge with potion. Fasten a cupping-glass to the belley, with a great fume, and also the navel, especially of the swelling be flatulent; make an issue on the inside of each leg, an handbreadth below the knee. Take specierum, diambræ diamolet, diacalaminti, diacinamoni, diocimini, and troch. de myrrh, of each two drams, sugar one pound: with betony water make lozenges: take of them two hours before meals. Apply to the bottom of the belly, as hot as may be endured, a little bag of camomile, cummin, and melilot, boiled in oil of rue; anoint the belly and secret parts with unguent agrippa and unguent arragons; mingle therewith oil of iros; cover the lower parts of the belly with the plaisters of bay berries, or a cataplasm made of cummin, camomile, briony roots, adding cow's and goat's dung.

Our moderns ascribe great virtues to tobacco-water distilled, and poured into the womb by a metrenchyta. Take hin, balm, southern-wood, origan, wormwood, calamint, bay leaves, marjoram, of each one handful; juniper berries four drams, with water make a decoction: of this may be made fomentations and infusions; make pessaries of storax, aloes, with the roots of dictau, aristolochia, and gentian. Instead of this you may use pessary, prescribed chapter xvii. Let her take of electuarium aromaticum, dissatyron, and eringo roots candied, every morning.

The air must be hot and dry; moderate exercise is allowed; much sleep is forbidden. She may eat the flesh of partridges, larks, chickens, mountain birds, hares, conies, &c. Let her drink be thin wine.

CHAPTER XI.

Of Moles and False Conceptions.

This disease is called by the Greeks mole; and the cause of this denomination is taken from the load or heavy weight of it, it being a mole, or great lump of hard flesh burdening the womb.

It is defined to be an inarticulate piece of flesh, without form, begotten in a matrix as if it were a true conception. In which definition we are to note two things: first, in that a mole is said to be inarticulate and without form, it differs from monsters, which are both formate and articulate: secondly, it is said to be as it were a true conception, which puts a difference between a true conception and a mole: which difference holds good three ways: first, in the genus, in that a mole cannot be said to be an animal: secondly, in the species, because it hath no human figure, and bears not the character of a man: thirdly, in the individual, for it hath no affinity with the parent, either in the whole body or any particular part of the same.

Cause. About the cause of this effect, among learned authors, I find a variety of judgments. Some are of opinion, that if the woman's seed goes into the womb, and not the man's, thereby is the mole produced. Others there be that affirm, it is engendered of the menstruous blood. But if these two were granted, then maids, by having their courses, or through nocturnal pollutions, might be subject to the same, which never yet any were. The true cause of this fleshy mole proceeds both from the man and from the woman, from corrupt and barren seed in man, and from the menstruous blood in the woman, both emitted together in the cavity of the womb, where nature finding herself weak, (yet desiring to maintain the perpetuity of her species,) labours to bring forth a vicious conception rather than none: and instead of a living creature, generates a lump of flesh.

Signs. The signs of a mole are these: the months are

suppressed, the appetite is depraved, the breasts swell, and the belly is suddenly puffed up, and waxeth hard. Thus far the signs of a breeding woman, and one that beareth a mole, are all one. I will show you how they differ. The first sign of difference is taken from the motion of a mole; it may be felt to move in the womb before the third month, which an infant cannot; yet the motion cannot be understood of any intelligent power in the mole, but the faculty of the womb and the animal spirits diffused through the substance of the mole; for it hath not an animal but a vegitative life, in manner of a plant: secondly, if a mole, the belly is suddenly puffed up; but if a true conception, the belly is suddenly retracted, and then riseth up by degrees: thirdly, the belly being pressed with the hand, the mole gives way; and the hand being taken away, it returns to the place again; but a child in the womb, though pressed with the hand, moves not presently; and being removed, returns slowly, or not at all; lastly, the child continues in the womb not above eleven months, but a mole continues sometimes four or five years, more or less, according as it is fastened in the matrix. I have known a mole fall away in four or five months. If it remain until the eleventh month, the legs wax feeble, and the whole body consumes, only the swelling of the belly still increases, which makes some think they are dropsical, though there be little reason for it; for in the dropsy the legs swell and grow big, but in a mole they consume and wither.

PROGNOSTICS. If, at the delivery of a mole, the flux of the blood be great, it shows the more danger, because the parts of nutrition having been violated by the flowing back of the superfluous humours, where the natural heat is consumed; and then parting with so much of her blood, the woman thereby is so weakened in all her faculties, that she cannot subsist without difficulty.

CURE. We are taught in the school of Hippocrates, that phlebotomy causeth abortion, by taking all that nourishment which should preserve the life of the child; wherefore, that this vicious conception may be deprived of that vegitative sap by which it lives, open the liver-vein and the saphena in both the feet, fasten cupping glasses to the loins and sides of the belly, which done, let the uterine parts be first mollified, and then the expulsive faculty provoked to expel the burden.

To laxate the ligature of the mole, take mallows with the roots, three handsfull; camomile, melilot, pelitory of the wall, violet leaves, mercury, root of fennel, parsley, of each two handsfull; linseed, fenugreek, each one pound; boil them in water, and let her sit therein up to the navel. At her going out of the bath, anoint the privates and reins with the following unguent: take oil of camomile, lilies, sweet almonds, one ounce each; fresh butter, laudanum, ammoniac, of each half an ounce: with the oil of linseed make an unguent. Or, instead of this may be used unguentum agrippa, or dialthea. Take mercury and althea roots, of each half a handful: flos, brachoc, ursini, half a handful; linseed, barley meal, of each six ounces; boil all these with water and honey, and make a plaister; make pessaries of the gum galbanum, bdellium, antimoniacum, figs, hog's suet, and honey.

After the ligaments of the mole are loosed, let the expulsive faculty be stirred up to expel the mole; for effecting of which all medicaments may be used which are proper to bring down the courses. Take troch. de myrrh one ounce; castor astrolochia, gentium, dictam, of each half an ounce; make a powder; take one dram in four ounces of mugwort water. Take of hypericon, calamint, pennyroyal, betony, hyssop, sage, horehound, valeria, madder, savine; with warer make a decoction: take three ounces of it, with one ounce and a half of feverfew. Take of mugwort, myrrh, gentian, pill. coch. of each four scruples; rue, pennyroyal, sage, panum, oppopanax, of each a dram; assafœtida, cinnamon, juniper berries, borage, of each one dram; with the juice of savine make pills to be taken every morning; make an infusion of hyssop, bay leaves, asirum, calamint; bay berries, camomile, mugwort, ervine, cloves, nutmeg, of each two scruples; galbanum one dram; hiera picra and black hellebore oil, of each one scruple; with turpentine make a pessary.

But if these things prove not available, then must the mole be drawn away with an instrument put up into the womb, called a pes griphus, which may be done with no great danger, if it be performed by a skilful surgeon. After the delivery of the mole, by reason that the woman hath parted with much blood already, let the flux of blood be stayed as soon as may be. Fasten cupping-glasses to the shoulders and ligatures to the arms. If this help not, open the liver vein in the right arm.

The air must be tolerably hot and dry, and dry diet, such as doth mollify and attenuate; she may drink white wine,

CHAPTER XII.

Of Conception; and how a Woman may know whether she hath conceived or not, and whether Male or a Female.

The natural instinct that nature has implanted in men and women to propagate their own species, puts them upon making use of those ways that nature has ordained for that end, which, after they have made use of, the woman many times, through ignorance of her having conceived, or want of that due care which she ought to take, is little better than a murderer of her own child, though she intends it not; for, after conception, finding herself not well, and, through ignorance, not knowing what is the matter with her, goes to a doctor and inquires of him: and he knowing nothing but what they tell him, and not thinking of their being with child, gives them strong cathartical potions which destroy the conception. And some there are, that out of a foolish coyness, though they do know they have conceived, yet will not confess it, that they might be instructed how to order themselves accordingly; those that are so coy may in time learn to be wiser; and for the sake of those that are ignorant, I shall set down the signs of conception, that women may thereby know whether they have conceived or not.

Signs. If under the eye the vein be swelled, that is, under the lower eyelid, the veins in the eyes appearing clearly, and the eyes sometimes discoloured, if the woman has not the terms upon her, nor watched the night before, you may certainly conclude her to be with child; and this appears most plainly just upon her conception; and the first two months I never knew this sign to fail.

Keep the urine of the woman close in a glass three days, and then strain it through a fine linen cloth : if you find small living creatures in it, she has most assuredly conceived with child; for the urine which was before part of her own substance, will be generated as well as its mistress.

A coldness and chillness of the outward parts after copulation, the heat being retired to make conception.

The veins of the breast are more clearly seen than they were wont to be.

The body is weakened, and the face discoloured.

The belly waxeth very flat, because the womb closeth itself together to nourish and cherish the seed.

If cold water be drank, a coldness is left in the breasts.

Loss of appetite to victuals, sour belchings, and exceeding weakness of stomach.

The breasts begin to swell and wax hard, not without pain and soreness.

Wringing or griping pains, like the cramp, happen in the belly about the navel.

Divers appetites and longings are engendered.

The veins of the eyes are clearly seen, and the eyes seem somewhat discoloured, as a looking glass will show you. This is an infallible sign.

The excrements of the guts are voided painfully, because the womb swelling thrusteth the right gut together.

Take a handsome green nettle, and put it into the urine of the woman; cover it close, and let it remain a whole night; if the woman be with child, it will be full of red spots on the morrow; if she be not, it will be blackish.

There are several other rules of this nature, but these are the best, and some of them seldom fail.

Now, because many are mighty desirous to know whether they be with child of a male or a female, I will in the next place lay down some rules whereby you may form a proper judgment in that case.

Signs of a Male Child.

The woman breeds a boy easier and with less pain than girls, and carries her burden not so heavily, but is more nimble in stirring.

The child is first felt by her on the right side; for the ancients are of opinion that male children lie on the right side of the womb. The woman, when she riseth up from a chair, doth sooner stay herself upon her right hand than on her left.

The belly lies rounder and higher than when it is a female.

The right breast is more plump and harder than the left, and the right nipple redder.

The colour of a woman is more clear and not so swarthy as when she conceives a girl.

The contrary to these are signs of the conception of a female, and therefore it is needless to say any thing of them.

But I will add the following, which have been the result of my own experience, and which I never knew to fail.

If the circle under the woman's eyes, which is of a wan blue colour, be more apparent under the right eye, and the veins most apparent in her right eye, and there most discoloured, she is with child of a boy; if the marks be most apparent in her left eye, she is with child of a girl.

Again, let her milk a drop of her milk in a basin of fair water; if it sinks to the bottom, as it drops in, round in a drop, it is a girl she is with child of; but if it be a boy, it will spread and swim at the top. This I have often tried, and it never failed.

CHAPTER XIII.

Of Untimely Births.

WHEN the fruit of the womb comes forth before the seventh month, that is, before it comes to maturity, it is said to be abortive; and, in effect, the child proves abortive (I mean, does not live) if born in the eighth month. And why children born in the seventh or ninth month may live, and not in the eighth month, may seem strange, yet it is ture. The cause thereof, by some, is ascribed to the planet under which the child is born; for every month, from the conception to the birth, is governed by its proper planet; and in the eighth month Saturn doth predominate, which is cold and dry; and coldness being an utter enemy to life, destroys the nature of the child. Hippocrates gives a better reason, viz. the infant being every way perfect and complete in the seventh month, desires more air and nutriment than it had before and because it cannot obtain these, it labours for a passage to go out: and if its spirits become weak and faint, and have not strength sufficient to break the membranes and come forth, as is decreed by nature, it shall continue in the womb till the ninth month, that in that time its wearied spirits may again be strengthened and refreshed; but if it returns to strive again the eighth month, and be born, it cannot live, because the day of its birth is either past or to come. For, in the eighth month, saith Aven, he is weak an infirm; and, therefore, being then cast into the cold air, his spirits cannot be supported.

CURE. Untimely birth may be caused by cold; for as it maketh the fruit of the tree to wither and to fall down before it be ripe, so doth it nip the fruit of the womb before it comes to full perfection, and makes it to be abortive: sometimes by humidity, weakening the faculty, that the fruit cannot be restrained till the due time: by dryness or emptiness, defrauding the child of its nourishment: by one of these alcine fluxes, by phlebotomy, and other evacuations: by inflammations of the womb, and other sharp diseases. Sometimes it is caused by joy, laughter, anger, and especially fear; for in that the heat forsakes the womb, and runs to the heart for help there, and so cold strikes in the matrix, whereby the ligaments are ralaxed, and so abortion follows; wherefore Plato, in his time, commanded that the women should shun all temptations of immoderate joy and pleasure, and likewise avoid all occasions of fear and grief. Abortion also may be caused by the corruption of the air, by filthy odours, and especially by the snuff of a candle; also by falls, blows, violent exercise, leaping, dancing, &c.

SIGNS. Signs of future abortion are, extenuation of the breasts, with a flux of watery milk, pain in the womb, heaviness in the head, unusual weariness in the hips and thighs, flowing of the courses. Signs foretelling the fruit to be dead in the womb, are hollowness in the eyes, pain in the head, anguish, horror, paleness of the face and lips, gnawing of the stomach, no motion of the infant, coldness and looseness of the mouth of the womb, and thickness of the belly, and watery and bloody excrements come from the matrix.

CHAPTER XIV.

Directions for Breeding Women.

The prevention of untimely births consists in taking away the forementioned causes, which must be effected before and after the conception.

Before conception, if the body be over hot, dry, or moist, correct it with the contraries: if couchmical, purge it; if phletorical, open the liver vein; if too gross, attenuate it; if too lean, corroborate and nourish it. All diseases of the womb must be removed as I have showed.

After conception, let the air be temperate; sleep not overmuch, avoid watchings, much exercise of body, passions of the mind, loud clamours, and filthy smells; sweet odours also are to be rejected of those that are hysterical. Abstain from all things which provoke either the urine or courses; also from salt, sharp, and windy meats. A moderate diet should be observed.

If the excrement of the guts be retained, lenify the belly with clysters made of the decoction of mallows, violets, with sugar and common oil: or make broth with borage, bugloss, beets, mallows, taking in the same a little manna. On the contrary if she be troubled with looseness in the belly, let it not be stayed without the judgment of a physician; for all the uterine fluxes have a malign quality in them, which must be evacuated before the flux be stayed.

The cough is another accident which accompanieth breeding women, and puts them in great danger of miscarrying, by a continual distillation falling from the brain. To prevent which, shave away the hair on the cornal and satical coissures, and apply thereon the following plaister: take of resinæ half an ounce, of laudana one dram, citron peel. lign, aloes, olibani, of each a dram; stirachis liquidæ, and sicca, a sufficient quantity; dissolve the gums in vinegar, and make a plaister: at night going to bed let her take the fume of these trochisks cast upon the coals. Also, take of frankincense, storax powder, and red roses, of each a dram and a half, sandrach eight drams, mastic, benjamin, amber, of each one dram; with turpentine make trochisks, apply a cautery to the nape of the neck, and every night let her take these pills following: take hypocistides, terriæ, sigillate, fine bole, of each half an ounce; bastort. alcatia, styracis, calamint, of each two drams, cloves one dram; with syrup of myrtles make pills.

In breeding women there is a corrupted matter generated, which flowing to the ventricle dejecteth the appetite, and causeth a vomiting; and the stomach being weak, and not able to digest this matter, sometimes sends it to the guts, whereby is caused a flux in the belly, which greatly stirreth up the faculty of the womb. To prevent all these dangers, the stomach must be corroborated as follows: take lign, aloes and nutmeg, of each one dram; mace, clove, mastic, and laudanum, of each two scruples; oil of spike an ounce; musk two grains; oil of mastic, quinces, and wormwood, of each half an ounce; make an unguent for the stomach to be applied before meals. But instead thereof may be used ceronum, stomachile, galeni. Take of conserve of borage, bugloss, and atthos. of each half an ounce; confect. de hyacinth, lemon peel candied, specierum, diamarg, pulv de gemmis, of each two drams; nutmeg and diambra, of each two scruples; piony roots and diacorati, of each two drams; with syrup of roses make an electuary; of which she must take twice a day two hours before meals. Another accident which perplexeth a woman with child is swelling of the legs, which happens the first three months, by superfluous humours falling down from the stomach and liver: for the cure whereof, take oil of roses two drams, salt and vinegar, of each one dram: shake them together until the salt be dissolved, and anoint the legs therewith hot, chafing it in with the hand: it may be done without danger in the fourth, fifth, or sixth month of pregnancy; for the child in the womb may be compared to an apple on a tree; the first three months it is weak and tender, subject, with the apple, to fall away; but afterwards, the membranes being strengthened, the fruit remains firmly fastened to the womb, not apt to mischances, and so continues until the seventh month, till growing near the time its ligaments are again relaxed, like the apple that is almost ripe, and grow looser every day until the fixed time of delivery. If, therefore, the body is in real need of purging, she may do it without danger in the fourth, fifth, or sixth months: but not before nor after, unless in some sharp diseases, in which the mother and the child both are like to perish. Apply plaisters and unguents to the reins, to strengthen the fruit of the womb. Take of gum agaric, galangale, bistort, hypocistic, and storax, of each one dram: fine bole, nutmeg, mastic, bollust, sanguis draconis, and myrtle berries, a dram and a half; wax and turpentine a sufficient quantity; make a plaister. Apply it to the reins in the winter time, and remove it every twenty-four hours, lest the reins be over hot therewith. In the interim anoint the privities and reins with unguent and consitissæ; but if it be the summer time, and the reins hot, the following plaister is more proper: take of red roses one pound, mastic and red sanders, of each two drams; bole ammoniac, red coral and bistort, each two drams; pomegranate peel prepared, and coriander, of each two drams and a half; barberries two scruples; oil of mastic and quinces, of each an ounce: juice of plantain two drams; with pitch make a plaister; anoint the reins also with unguentum sandal. Once every week wash the reins with two parts of rose water, and one part of white wine mingled together and warmed at the fire. This will assuage the heat of the reins, and disperse the oil of the plaister out of the pores of the skin, and cause the ointment or plaister the sooner to penetrate and strengthen the womb. Some are of opinion, that as long as the loadstone is laid to the navel, it keeps the woman from abortion. The like is also recorded of the stone ætites, being hanged about the neck; the same virtue hath the stone samlus.

CHAPTER XV.

Directions to be observed by Women at the time of their falling in Labour, in order to their safe Delivery, with Directions for Midwives.

HAVING given necessary directions for child-bearing women, how to govern themselves during the time of their pregnancy, I shall add what is necessary for them to observe in order to their delivery.

The time of birth drawing near, let the woman be careful to send for a skilful midwife, and that rather too soon than too late; against which time let her prepare a pallet, bed, or couch, and place it near the fire, that the midwife and her assistants may pass round, and help on every side as occasion requires, having a change of linen ready, and a small stool to rest her feet against, she having more force when they are bowed than when they are otherwise.

Having thus provided, when the woman feels her pain come, and the weather not cold, let her walk about the room, resting herself by turns upon the bed, and so expect the coming down of her water, which is a humour contracted in one of the outward membranes, and flows thence when it is broke by the struggling of the child, there being no direct time fixed for the efflux, though generally it flows not above two hours before the birth. Motion will likewise cause the womb to open and dilate itself, when from lying long in bed it is uneasy. Yet if she be very weak, she may take some gentle cordial to refresh herself, if her pain will permit.

If her travail be tedious, she may revive her spirits with taking chicken or mutton broth, or she may take a poached egg, but must take heed of eating to excess.

As for the postures women are delivered in, there are many, some lying on their beds, some sitting in a chair, supported and held by others, or resting upon the bed or chair; some again upon their knees, being supported upon their arms; but the most safe and commodious way is in the bed, and then the midwife ought to mind the following rules:—Let her lay the woman upon her back, her head a little raised by the help of a pillow, having the like help to support her reins and buttocks, and that the rump may lie high: for if she lies low, she cannot well be delivered. Then let her keep her knees and thighs as far distant as she can, her legs bowed together to her buttocks, the soles of her feet and heels being fixed upon a little log of timber placed for that purpose, that she may strain the stronger; and in case her back be very weak, a swathing band must be cast under it, the band being four times double, and about two inches broad; and this must be held by two persons, who with steady hands and equal motion must raise her up at the time her pains happen; but if they be not exact in their motion, it is better to let it alone. And at the same time, let two women hold her shoulders that she may then strain out the birth with more advantage; and then, to facilitate it, let a woman stroke or press the upper part of the belly gently and by degrees. Nor must the woman herself be faint hearted, but of good courage, forcing herself by straining and holding her breath.

In case of delivery, the midwife must wait with patience till the child's head or other members burst the membrane; for if through ignorance, or haste to go to other women, as some have done, the midwife tear the membrane with her nails, she endangers both the woman and the child; for by lying dry, and wanting that slipperiness that should make it easy, it comes forth with great pains.

When the head appears, the midwife must gently hold it between her hands, and draw the child at such times as the woman's pains are upon her, and at no other, slipping by degrees her forefingers under its arm pits, not using a rough hand in drawing it forth, lest by that means the tender infant may receive any deformity of body. As soon as the child is taken forth, which is for the most part with its face downwards, let it be laid on its back, that it may more freely receive external respiration; then cut the navel string about three inches from the body, tying that end which adheres to the body with a silken string, as near as you can; then cover the head and stomach of the child well, suffering nothing to come upon the face.

The child being thus brought forth, if healthy lay it by, and let the midwife regard the patient in drawing forth the secundine; and this she may do by wagging and stirring them up and down, and afterwards with a gentle hand drawing them forth; and if the work be difficult, let the woman hold salt in her hands, shut them close, and breathe hard into them, and hereby she will know whether the membranes be broken or not. It may be also known by causing her to strain or vomit, by putting her finger down her throat, or by straining or moving her lower parts; but let all be done out of hand. If this fail, let her take a draught of raw elder water, or yolk of a new laid egg, and smell to a piece of assafœtida. especially if she is troubled with the windy cholic. If she happen to take cold, it is a great obstruction to the coming down of the secundine; and in such cases, the midwife ought to chafe the woman's belly gently, to break not only the wind, but oblige the secundine to come down. But these proving ineffectual, the midwife must insert her hand into the extern or orifice of the womb, and gently draw it forth.

Having now discoursed of common births, or such as for the most part are easy, I shall now give directions in cases of extremity.

CHAPTER XVI.

In Case of Extremity, what ought to be observed; especially to Women, who, in their Travail, are attended with a Flux of Blood, Convulsions and Fits of the Mind.

If the woman's labour be hard and difficult, greater regard must be had then at other times.—And first of all, the situation of the womb and posture of lying must be across the bed, being held by strong persons to prevent her slipping down or moving herself in the operation of the chirurgeon; her thighs must be put asunder, as far distant as may be, and so held; whilst her head must lean upon a bolster, and the reins of her back be supported after the same manner. Her rump and buttocks being lifted up, observe to cover her stomach, belly, and thighs, with warm linen, to keep them from the cold.

The woman being in this posture, let the operator put up his or her hand, if the neck of the womb be dilated, and remove the contracted blood that obstructs the passage of the birth; and having by degrees gently made way, let him tenderly move the infant, his hand being first anointed with sweet butter or a harmless pomatum. And if the waters be not come down, then without difficulty may they be let forth; when, if the infant should attempt to break out with its head foremost, or cross, he may gently turn it to find the feet; which having done, let him draw forth the one, and fasten it to the riband, then put it up again, and by degrees find the other, bringing them as close and even as may be, and between whiles let the woman breathe, urging her to strain, in helping nature to perfect the birth, that it may be drawn forth; and the readier to do it, and that the hold may be the surer, wrap a linen cloth about the child's thighs, observing to bring it into the world with its face downwards.

In case of a flux of blood, if the neck of the womb be open, it must be considered whether the infant or secundine comes first, which the latter sometimes happening to do, stops the mouth of the womb, and hinders the birth, endangering both the woman and child; but in this case the secundine must be removed by a swift turn; and indeed they have by their so coming down deceived many, who feeling their softness, supposed the womb was not dilated, and by this means the woman and child, or at least the latter, has been lost. The secundine moved, the child must be sought for, and drawn forth, as has been directed; and if in such a case the woman or child die, the midwife or surgeon is blameless, because they did their true endeavour.

If it appears upon inquiry that the secundine comes first, let the woman be delivered with all convenient expedition, because a great flux of blood will follow; for the veins are opened, and upon this account two things are to be considered.

First, The manner of the secundine advancing, whether it be much or little. If the former, and the head of the child appear first, it may be guided and directed towards the neck of the womb, as in the case of natural birth; but if there appear any difficulty in the delivery, the best way is to search for the feet, and thereby draw it forth: but if the latter, the secundine may be put back with a gentle hand, and the child first taken forth.

But if the secundine be far advanced, so that it cannot be put back, and the child follow it close, then is the secundine to be taken forth with much care, as swift as may be, and laid easy without cutting the entrail that is fastened to them; for thereby you may be guided to the infant, which, whether alive or dead, must be drawn forth by the feet in all haste; though it is not to be acted unless in case of great necessity, for in other cases the secundine ought to come last.

And in drawing forth a dead child, let these directions be carefully observed by the surgeon, viz. If the child be found dead, its head being foremost, the delivery will be more difficult; for it is an apparent sign, by the woman's strength beginning to fail her, that the child, being dead, and wanting its natural force, can be no ways assisting to its delivery; wherefore the most certain and safe way for the surgeon is to put up his left hand, sliding it as hollow in the palm as he can into the neck of the womb, and into the lower part thereof towards the feet, and then between the head of the infant and the neck of the matrix; then having a hook in the right hand, couch it close, and slip it up above the left hand, between the head of the child and the flat of his hand, fixing it in the bars of the temple towards the eye. For want of a convenient coming at these in the occiputal bone, observe still to keep the left hand in its place, and with it gently moving and stirring the head, and so with the right hand and hook draw the child forward, admonishing the woman to put forth her utmost strength, still drawing when the woman's pangs are upon her. The head being drawn out, with all speed he must slip his hand up under the arm-holes of the child, and take it quite out; giving these things to the woman, viz. a toast of fine wheaten bread in a quarter of a pint of Ipocras wine.

Now the former application failing, when the woman is in her bed, let her receive the following portion hot, and rest till she feels the operation.

Take seven blue figs, cut them to pieces, add to them fenugreek, motherwort, and seed of rue, of each five drams; water of Pennyroyal and motherwort, of each six ounces; boil them till one half be consumed; and having strained them again, add trochisks of myrrh one dram, and saffron three grains; sweeten the liquor with loaf sugar, and spice it with cinnamon.

Having rested upon this, let her labour again as much as may be: and if she be not successful make a fumigation of castor, opopanax, and sulphur, and assafœdita, of each half a dram, beating them into powder, and wetting them with the juice of rue, so that the smoke or fume may only come to the matrix, and no further.

If these effect not your desire, then the following plaister is to be applied, viz. Take of galbanum an ounce and a half; colocynthia without grains, two drams; the juice of motherwort and rue, of each half an ounce, add seven ounces of virgin bees' wax: bruise and melt them together, spreading them on a searcloth, to reach from the navel to the os pubis, spreading also the flax, at the same time making a convenient pessary of wood, closing it in a bag of silk, and dipping it in a decoction of round birthwort, savin, colocynthia with grains; stavescare, black hellebore, of each one dram; a little sprig of rue.

But those things not having the desired success, and the woman's danger still increasing, let the surgeon use his instrument to dilate and widen the womb; to which end the woman must be set in a chair, so that she may turn her crupper as much from its back as is convenient. drawing likewise her legs up as close as she can, spreading her thighs as wide as may be: or if she be very weak, it may be more convenient that she be laid on a bed with her head downwards, and her buttocks raised, and both legs drawn up as much as may be; the surgeon then, with his speculum matricis, or his apertory, may dilate the womb, and draw out the child and secundine together, if it be possible: the whole being done, the womb must be well washed and anointed, and the woman laid in her bed, and comforted with spices and cordials. This course must be taken in the delivery of all dead children, likewise with moles, secundines, and false births, that will not of themselves come forth in season. If the instrument aforesaid will not sufficiently widen the womb, then other instruments, as the drake's bill, and long pincers, ought to be used.

If it so happen that any inflammation, swelling, or congealed blood be contracted in the matrix, under the film of these tumours, either before or after the birth, where the matter appears thinner, then let the midwife, with a penknife, or incision instrument, lance it, and press out the corruption, healing it with a pessary dipt in oil of red roses.

If at any time through cold or some violence, the child happens to be swelled in any part, or hath contracted a watery humour, if it remain alive, such means must be used as are least injurious to the child or mother: but if it be dead, the humours must be let out by incision to facilitate the birth.

If, as it often happens, that the child comes with its feet foremost, and the hands dilating themselves from the hips, in such cases the midwife must be provided with necessary instruments to stroke and anoint the infant with, to help it coming forth. lest it turn again into the womb, holding at the same time both the arms of the infant close to the hips, that so it may issue forth after this manner; but if it proves too big, the womb must be well anointed. The woman must also take sneezing-powder, to make her strain; those who attend may gently stroke her belly to make the birth descend, and keep it from retiring back.

Sometimes it falls out, that the child coming with the feet foremost has its arms extended above its head; but the midwife must not receive it so, but put it back into the womb, unless the passages be extraordinarily wide, and then she must anoint both the child and the womb: nor is it safe so to draw it forth, which must be done after this manner: the woman must be laid on her back, with her head depressed, and her buttocks raised: and then the midwife, with a gentle hand, must compress the belly of the womb, by that means to put back the infant, observing to turn the face of the child towards the back of its mother, raising up its thighs and buttocks towards her navel, that so the birth may be mo natural

If a child happen to come forth with one foot, the arm being extended along the side, and the other foot turned backward. then must the woman be instantly taken to her bed, and laid in the posture above described, at which time the midwife must carefully put back the foot so appearing. and the woman rock herself from one side to the other, till she find the child is turned, but must not alter the posture, nor turn upon her face; after which she may expect her pains, and must have great assistance and cordials to revive and support her spirits.

At other times it happens that the child lies across in the womb, and falls upon its side: in this case the woman must not be urged in her labour, neither can any expect the birth in such a manner: therefore the midwife, when she finds it so, must use great diligence to reduce it to its right form, or at least to such a form in the womb as may make the delivery possible and most easy, by moving the buttocks, and guiding the head to the passage: and if she be unsuccessful herein, let the woman again try by rocking herself to and fro, and wait with patience till it alters its manner of lying.

Sometimes the child hastens the birth, by expanding its legs and arms; in which, as in the former case, the woman must rock herself, but not with violence, till she finds those parts fall to their proper stations; or it may be done by a gentle compression of the womb; but if neither of them prevail, the midwife, with her hand, must close the legs of the infant; and, if she come at them, do the like to the arms, and so draw it forth: but if it can be reduced of itself to the posture of a natural birth it is better.

If the infant comes forward with both knees foremost, and the hands hanging down upon the thighs, then must the midwife put both knees upward, till the feet appear; taking hold of which with her left hand, let her keep her right hand on the side of the child, and in that posture endeavour to bring it forth. But if she cannot do this, then also must the woman rock herself till the child is in a more convenient posture for delivery.

Sometimes it happens that the child presses forward with one arm stretched on its thighs, and the other raised over its head, and the feet stretched out at length in the womb. In such case, the midwife must not attempt to receive the child in that posture, but must lay the woman on the bed in the manner aforesaid, making a soft and gentle compression on her belly, to oblige the child to retire; which, if it does not, then must the midwife thrust it back by the shoulder, and bring the arm that was stretched above the head to its right station: for there is more danger in these extremities: and, therefore the midwife must anoint her hands and the womb of the woman with sweet butter, or a proper pomatum, and thrust her hand as near as she can to the arm of the infant, and bring it to the side. But if this cannot be done, let the woman be laid on her bed to rest awhile: in which time, perhaps, the child may be reduced to a better posture: which the midwife finding, she must draw tenderly the arms close to the hips, and so receive it.

If an infant come with its buttocks foremost, and almost double, the midwife must anoint her hand and thrust it up, and gently heaving up the buttocks and back, strive to turn the head to the passage, but not too hastily, lest the infant's retiring should shape it worse; and, therefore, if it cannot be turned with the hand, the woman must rock herself on the bed, taking such comfortable things as may support her spirits, till she perceives the child to turn.

If the child's neck be bowed, and it comes forward with its shoulders, as sometimes it doth, with the hands and feet stretched upwards, the midwife must gently move the shoulders, that she may direct the head to the passage; and the better to effect it, the woman must rock herself as aforesaid.

These and other the like methods are to be observed in case a woman hath twins, or three children at a birth, which sometimes happens: for, as the single birth hath but one natural and many unnatural forms, even so it may be in a double or treble birth.

Wherefore, in all such cases, the midwife must take care to receive that first which is nearest the passage: but not letting the other go, lest by retiring it should change the form; and when one is born, she must be speedy in bringing forth the other. And this birth, if it be in the natural way, is more easy, because the children are commonly less than those of single birth, and so require a less passage. But if this birth come unnaturally, it is far more dangerous than the other.

In the birth of twins, let the widwife be very careful that the secundine be naturally brought forth, lest the womb, being delivered of its burden, fall, and so the secundine continue longer there than is consistent with the woman's safety.

But if one of the twins happen to come with the head, the other with the feet foremost, then let the midwife deliver the natural birth first; and if she cannot turn the other, draw it out in the posture it presses forward: but if that with its feet downward be foremost, she may deliver that first, turning the other side. But in this case the midwife must carefully see that it be not a monstrous birth, instead of twins, a body with two heads, or two bodies joined together, which she may soon know; if both the heads come foremost, by putting up her hand between them, as high as she can; and then, if she find they are twins, she may gently put one of them aside to make way for the other, taking that first which is most advanced, leaving the other so that it do not change its situation. And, for the safety of the other child, as soon as it comes forth out of the womb, the midwife must tie the navel string, as hath before been directed; and also bind, with a large and long fillet, that part of the navel that is fastened to the secundine the more readily to find it.

The second infant being born, let the midwife carefully examine whether there be not two secundines; for some times it falls out, that by the shortness of the ligament, it retires back to the prejudice of the woman. Wherefore, lest the womb should close, it is most expedient to hasten them forth with all convenient speed.

If two infants are joined together by the body, as sometimes it monstrously falls out, then, though the head should come foremost, yet it is proper, if possible, to turn them, and draw them forth by the feet, observing, when they come to the hips, to draw them out as soon as may be. And here great care ought to be used in anointing and widening the passage. But these sorts of births rarely happening, I need to say the less of them: and, therefore, shall next show how women should be ordered after delivery.

CHAPTER XVII.

How Childbearing Women ought to be ordered after Delivery.

If a woman has had very hard labour, it is necessary she should be wrapped up in a sheep's skin, taken off before it is cold, applying the fleshy side to her reins or belly: or, for want of this, the skin of a hare or coney, flayed off as soon as killed, may be applied to the same parts: and in so doing, a dilation being made in the birth, and the melancholy blood expelled in these parts, continue these for an hour or two.

Let the woman afterwards be swathed with fine linen cloth, about a quarter of a yard in breadth, chafing her belly, before it is swathed, with oil of St. John's wort; after that, raise up the matrix with a linen cloth, many times folded, then with a linen pillow or quilt, cover her flanks, and place the swathe somewhat above the haunches, winding it pretty stiff, applying at the same time, a warm cloth to her nipples; do not immediately use the remedies to keep back the milk, by reason, the body at such a time, is out of frame; for there is neither vein nor artery which does not strongly beat: and remedies to drive back the milk, being of a dissolving nature, it is improper to apply them to the breasts, during such disorder, lest by doing so, evil humours be contracted in the breast. Wherefore, twelve hours at least ought to be allowed for the circulation and settlement of the blood, and what was cast on the lungs by the vehement agitation during the labour, to retire to its proper receptacles.

Some time after delivery, you may make a restrictive of the yolks of two eggs, and a quarter of a pint of white wine, oil of St. John's wort, oil of roses, plantain, and rose-water, of each one ounce; mix them together, fold a linen cloth, and apply it to the breast, and the pains of those parts will be greatly eased.

She must by no means sleep directly after delivery; but about four hours after, she may take broth, caudle, or such liquid victuals as are nourishing; and if she be disposed to sleep, it may be very safely permitted. And this is as much in case of a natural birth as ought immediately to be done.

But in case of an extremity, or an unnatural birth, the following rules ought to be observed:

In the first place, let the woman keep a temperate diet, by no means overcharging herself after such en extraordinary evacuation, not being ruled by giving credit to unskilful nurses, who admonish them to feed heartily, the better to repair the loss of blood. For that blood is not for the most part pure, but such as has been detained in the vessels or membrane, better voided, for the health of the woman, than kept, unless there happen an extraordinary flux of the blood. For if her nourishment be too much, it may make her liable to a fever, and increase the milk too much: which curding, very often turns to imposthumes.

Wherefore, it is requisite, for the first five days especially, that she take moderately, panado broth, poached eggs, jelly of chickens or calves' feet, or fresh barley broth, every day increasing the quantity a little.

And if she intend to be a nurse to her child, she must take something more than ordinary, to increase the milk by degrees, which must be of no continuance, but drawn off either by the child or otherwise. In this case likewise, observe to let her have coriander or fennel seeds boiled in barley broth; but by all means, for the time specified, let her abstain from meat. If no fever trouble her, she may drink now and then a small quantity of pure white wine or claret, as also, syrup of maiden-hair, or any other syrup that is of an astringent quality, taken in a little water well boiled.

After the fear of a fever or contraction of humour in the breast is over, she may be nourished more plentifully with the broth of pullets, capons, pigeons, mutton, veil, &c. which must not be till after eight days from the time of delivery: at which time the womb, unless some accident hinder, has purged itself. It will be then likewise expedient to give cold meats, but let it be sparingly, that so she may the better gather strength. And let her, during the time, rest quietly and free from disturbance, not sleeping in the day-time if she can avoid it.

Take of both the mallows and pellitory of the wall a handful: camomile and melilot flowers, of each a handful; anniseed and fennel seed, of each two ounces; boil them in a decoction of sheep's head, and take of this three quarts dissolving in it common honey, coarse sugar, and new fresh butter, two ounces; strain it well, and administer it clysterwise; but if it does not operate well, take an ounce of catholicon.

CHAPTER XVIII.

How to expel the Cholic from Women in Childbirth.

These pains frequently afflict the women no less than the pains of her labour, and are by the ignorant taken many times the one for the other: and sometimes they happen both at the same instant; which is occasioned by a raw, crude, and watery matter in the stomach, contracted through ill digestion; and while such pains continue, the woman's travail is retarded.

Therefore, to expel fits of cholic, take two ounces of oil of sweet almonds, and an ounce of cinnamon water, with three or four drops of spirits of ginger: then let the woman drink it off.

If this does not abate the pain, make a clyster of camomile, balm-leaves, oil of olives, and new milk, boiling the former in the latter. Administer it as is usual in such cases. And then fomentations proper for dispelling of wind will not be amiss.

If the pain produce a griping in the guts after-delivery, then take of the root of great comfrey one dram, nutmeg and peach kernels of each two scruples, yellow amber eight drams, ambergrease one scruple: bruise them together, and give them to the woman as she is laid down, in two or three spoonfuls of white wine: but if she be feverish, then let it be in as much warm broth.

THE FAMILY PHYSICIAN.

BEING

CHOICE AND APPROVED REMEDIES FOR SEVERAL DISTEMPERS INCIDENTAL TO HUMAN BODIES.

For the Apoplexy.

Take man's skull prepared, powder of the roots of male peony, of each an ounce and a half; contrayerva, bastard dittany, angelica, zedoary, of each two drams: mix and make a powder; add thereto two ounces of candied orange and lemon peel, beat all together to a powder, whereof you may take half a dram or a dram.

A Powder for the Epilepsy or falling Sickness

Take of opopanax, crude antimony, dragon's blood, castor, peony-seeds, of each an equal quantity; make a subtle powder: the dose, half a dram, in black cherry-water. Before you take it, the stomach must be cleansed with some proper vomit, as that of Mynficht's emetic tartar, from four grains to six: if for children, salt of vitriol, from a scruple to half a dram.

For a Head-ache of a long standing.

Take the juice of powder or distilled water of hog-lice, and continue the use of it.

For Spitting of Blood.

Take conserve of comfrey and of hips, of each an ounce and a half; conserve red roses, three ounces; dragon's blood, a dram; species of hyacinths, two scruples; red coral, a dram; mix, and with syrup of red poppies make a soft electuary. Take the quantity of a walnut night and morning.

For a Looseness.

Take Venice treacle and diascordium, of each half a dram, in warm ale or water-gruel, or what you like best at night going to bed.

For the Bloody-Flux.

First take a dram of powder of rhubarb, in a sufficient quantity of conserve of red roses, in the morning early: then at night, take of torrified or roasted rhubarb, half a dram; diascordium, a dram and a half: liquid laudanum cydomated, a scruple; mix, and make a bolus.

For an Inflammation of the Lungs.

Take of charious water, ten ounces; water of red poppies, three ounces: syrup of poppies, an ounce: pearl prepared, a dram: make a julep, and take a spoonful every fourth hour.

Ointment for the Pleurisy.

Take of oil of violets or sweet almonds, of each an ounce, with wax and a little saffron: make an ointment, warm it and bathe it upon the part affected.

An Ointment for the Itch.

Take sulphur vive in powder, half an ounce, oil of tartar per deliquium a sufficient quantity, ointment of roses four ounces: make a liniment, to which add a scruple of rhodium to aromatize, and rub the parts affected by it.

For a Running Scab.

Take two pounds of tar, incorporate it into a thick mass with well sifted ashes: boil the mass in fountain water, adding leaves of ground-ivy, white horehound, fumitory roots, sharp pointed dock, and of flocan pan, of each four handsfull: make a bath, to be used with care of taking cold.

For Worms in Children.

Take wormseed half a dram, flour of sulphur a dram, salt prunel half a dram: mix, and make a powder. Give as much as will lie on a silver three-pence, night and morning, in grocer's treacle or honey; or to people grown up, you may add a sufficient quantity of aloe rosatum, and so make them up into pills; three or four may be taken every morning.

For Fevers in Children.

Take crabs-eyes a dram, cream of tartar half a dram white sugar-candy finely powdered weight of both; mix all well together, and give as much as will lie on a silver three-pence, in a spoonful of barley-water or sack-whey.

A Quiet Night Draught when the Cough is violent.

Take water of green wheat six ounces, syrup diascordium three ounces, take two or three spoonsful going to bed every night, or every other night.

An Electuary for the Dropsy.

Take best rhubard one dram, gum lac prepared two drams, zyloaloes, cinnamon, long-birth worth, half an ounce each, best English saffron half a scruple; with a syrup of chychory and rhubard make an electuary. Take the quantity of a nutmeg or small walnut, every morning fasting.

For a Tympany Dropsy.

Take roots of cheveril and candied eringo roots half an ounce each, roots of butcher broom two ounces, grass-roots three ounces shaving of ivory and hartshorn two drams and a half each, burdock seeds three drams; boil them in two or three pounds of spring water. While the strained liquor is hot, pour it upon the leaves of water-cresses and goose-grass bruised, of each a handful, adding a pint of Rhenish wine. Make a close infusion for two hours, then strain out the liquor again, and add to it three ounces of magistral water and earth worms, and an ounce and a half of the syrup of the five opening roots. Make an apozem, whereof take four ounces twice a day.

For an Inward Bleeding.

Take leaves of plantain and stinging-nettles, of each three handfulls, bruise them well, and pour on them six ounces of plantain water, afterwards make a strong impression, and drink the whole off. Probatum est.

GENERAL OBSERVATIONS,

WORTHY OF NOTICE.

WHEN YOU FIND

A red man to be faithful, a tall man to be wise, a fat man to be swift of foot, a lean man to be a fool, a handsome man not to be proud, a poor man not to be envious, a knave to be no liar, an upright man not to bold and hearty to his own loss, one that drawls when he speaks not to be crafty and circumventing, one that winks on another with his eyes not to be false and deceitful, a sailor and hangman to be pitiful, a poor man to build churches, a quack doctor to have a good conscience, a bailiff not to be a merciless villain, an hostess not to over-reckon you, and an usurer to be charitable,

THEN SAY,

Ye have found a prodigy,
Men acting contrary to the common course of nature.

THE EXPERIENCED MIDWIFE.

INTRODUCTION.

I HAVE given this Book the title of The Experienced Midwife, both because it is chiefly designed for those that profess Midwifery, and contains whatever is necessary for them to know in the practice thereof: and also, because it is the result of many years' experience, and that in the most difficult cases, and is, therefore, the more to be depended upon.

A midwife is the most necessary and honourable office, being indeed a helper of nature: which therefore makes it necessary for her to be well acquainted with all the operations of nature in the work of generation, and instruments with which she works. For she that knows not the operations of nature, nor with what tools she works, must needs be at a loss how to assist therein. And seeing the instruments of operation, both in men and women, are those things by which mankind is produced, it is very necessary that all Midwives should be well acquainted with them, that they may the better understand their business, and assist nature as there shall be occasion.

The first thing then necessary as introductory to this treatise is an anatomical description of the several parts of generation both in men and women; but, as in the former part of this work, I have treated at large upon these subjects, being desirous to avoid tautology, I shall not here repeat any thing of what was then said, but refer the reader thereto, as a necessary introduction to what follows. And though I shall be necessitated to speak plainly, that so I may be understood, yet I shall do it with that modesty, that none shall have need to blush, unless it be from something in themselves, rather than from what they shall find here; having the motto of the royal garter for my defence, which is, "Honi soit qui mal y pense." "Evil be to him that evil thinks."

A GUIDE

TO

CHILD-BEARING WOMEN.

PART SECOND.

CHAPTER VIII.

SECTION I. *Of the Womb.*

IN this chapter I am to treat of the womb, which the Latins call matrix. Its parts are two; the mouth of the womb, and the bottom of it. The mouth is an orifice at the entrance into it, which may be dilated and shut together like a purse: for although in the act of copulation, it is big enough to receive the glands of the yard, yet, after conception, it is so close and shut that it will not admit the point of a bodkin to enter; and yet again, at the time of the woman's delivery, it is opened to such an extraordinary degree, that the infant passeth through it into the world: at which time this orifice wholly disappears, and the womb seems to have but one great cavity from its bottom to the entrance of the neck. When a woman is not with child, it is a little oblong, and of substance very thick and close; but when she is with child, it is shortened, and its thickness diminisheth proportionably to its distension: and therefore, it is a mistake of some anatomists, who affirm that its substance waxeth thicker a little before a woman's labour, for any one's reason will inform him, that the more distended it is, the thinner it must be; and the nearer a woman is to the time of her delivery, the shorter her womb must be extended. As to the action by which this inward orifice of the womb is opened and shut, it is purely natural; for, were it otherwise, there would not be so many bastards begotten as there are; nor would any married woman have so many children. Were it in their own power, they would hinder conception, though they would be willing enough to use copulation; for nature has attended that action with something so pleasing and delightful, that they are willing to indulge themselves in the use thereof, notwithstanding the pains they afterwards endure, and the hazard of their lives that often follows it. And this comes to pass, not so much from an inordinate lust in women, as that the great Director of Nature, for the increase and multiplication of mankind, and even of all other species in the elementary world, hath placed such a magnetic virtue in the womb, that it draws the seed to it as the loadstone does iron.

The Author of Nature has placed the womb in the belly, that the heat might always be maintained by the warmth of the parts surrounding it: it is therefore seated in the middle of the hypogastrum (or lower part of the belly,) between the bladder and the rectum (or right gut,) by which also it is defended from any hurt through the hardness of the bones: and it is placed in the lower part of the belly for the conveniency of copulation, and of a birth's being thrust out at the full time.

It is of a figure almost round, inclining somewhat to an oblong, in part resembling a pear; for, being broad at the bottom, it gradually terminates in the point of the orifice, which is narrow.

The length, breadth, and thickness of the womb differ according to the age and disposition of the body. For in virgins not ripe it is very small in all its dimensions; but, in women whose terms flow in great quantities, and such as frequently use copulation, it is much larger; and if they have had children, it is larger in them than in such as have had none; but, in women of a good stature, and well shaped, it is (as I have said before,) from the entry of the privy parts to the bottom of the womb, usually about eight inches, but the length of the body of the womb alone does not exceed three; the breadth thereof is near about the same, and of the thickness of the little finger, when the womb is not pregnant; but, when the woman is with child, it becomes of a prodigious greatness, and the nearer she is to her delivery the more is the womb extended.

It is not without reason then that nature (or the God of nature) has made the womb of a membranous substance; for thereby it does the easier open to conceive, is gradually dilated by the growth of the fœtus, or young one, and is afterwards contracted and closed again, to thrust forth both it and the afterburden, and then to retire to its primitive seat. Hence also it is enabled to expel any noxious humours which may sometimes happen to be contained within it.

Before I have done with the womb, which is the field of generation, and ought therefore to be the more particularly taken care of, (for as the seeds of plants can produce no plants, nor spring, unless sown in ground proper to awaken and excite their vegetative virtue, so likewise the seed of a man, though potentially containing all the parts of a child, never produce so admirable an effect, if it were not cast into the fruitful field of nature, the womb;) I shall proceed to a more particular description of its parts, and the uses for which nature hath designed them.

The womb then is composed of various similar parts, that is, of membranes, veins, arteries, and nerves. Its membranes are two, and they compose the principal parts of its body; the outermost of which ariseth from the peritoneum, or caul, and is very thin, without smooth, but within equal, that it may the better cleave to the womb, as it is fleshier and thicker than any thing else we meet within the body when the woman is not pregnant, and is interwoven with all sorts of fibres or small strings, that it may the better suffer the extension of the child and the waters caused during the pregnancy, and also that it may the easier close again after the delivery.

The veins and arteries proceed both from the hypogastrics and the spermatic vessels, of which I shall speak by and by; all these are inserted and terminated in the proper membrane of the womb. The arteries supply it with food for nourishment, which, being brought together in too great a quantity, sweats through the substance of it, and distils as it were a dew into the bottom of the cavity: from whence do proceed both the terms in ripe virgins, and the blood which nourisheth the embryo in breeding women. The branches which issue from the spermatic vessels are inserted in each side of the bottom of the womb, and are much less than those which proceed from the hypogastrics, those being greater, and bedewing the whole substance of it. There are yet some other small vessels, which arising the one from the other, are conducted to the internal orifice, and by these those that are pregnant do purge away the superfluity of their terms, when they happen to have more than is used in the nourishment of the infant: by which means nature hath taken such care of the womb, that during its pregnancy it shall not be obliged to open itself for the passing away those excrementitious humours, which, should it be forced to do, might often a danger abortion.

As touching the nerves, they proceed from the brain, which furnishes all the inner parts of the lower belly with them, which is the true reason it hath so great a sympathy with the stomach, which is likewise very considerably furnished from the same part: so that the womb cannot be afflicted with any pain but the stomach is immediately sensible thereof, which is the cause of those loathings or frequent vomitings which happen to it.

But, besides all these parts which compose the womb, it hath yet four ligaments, whose office it is to keep it firm in its place, and prevent its constant agitation, by the continual motion of the intestines which surround it; two of which are above, and two below. Those above are called the broad ligaments, because of their broad and membranous figure, and are nothing else but the production of the peritoneum, which, growing out of the side of the loins, towards the reins, come to be inserted in the sides of the bottom of the womb, to hinder the body from bearing too much on the neck, and so from suffering a precipitation, as will sometimes happen when the ligaments are too much relaxed; and do also contain the testicles, and as well safely conduct the different vessels as the ejaculatories to the womb. The lowermost are called round ligaments, taking their original from the side of the womb near the horn, from which they pass the groin, together with the production of the peritoneum, which accompanies them through the rings and holes of the oblique and transverse muscles of the belly, by which they divide themselves into many little branches, resembling the foot of a goose, of which some are inserted into the os pubis, and the rest are lost and confounded with the membranes that cover the upper and interior parts of the thigh: and it is that which causeth the numbness which women with child feel in their thighs. These two ligaments are long, round, and nervous, and pretty big in their beginning, near the matrix, hollow in their rise, and all along to the os pubis, where they are a little smaller, and become flat, the better to be inserted in the manner aforesaid. It is by their means the womb is hindered from rising too high. Now, although the womb is held in its natural situation by means of these four ligaments, yet it has liberty enough to extend itself when pregnant, because they are very loose, and so easily yield to distention. But, besides these ligaments, which keep the womb as it were in a poise, yet it is fastened, for greater security, by its neck, both to the bladder and rectum, between which it is situated.—Whence it comes to pass, that if at any time the womb be inflamed, it communicates the inflammation to the neighbouring parts.

Its use or proper action, in the work of generation, is to receive and retain the seed, and deduce from it power and action by its heat for the generation of the infant; and is therefore absolutely necessary for the conservation of the species. It also seems by accident to receive and expel the impurities of the whole body, as when women have abundance of whites; and to purge away, from time to time, the superfluity of the blood, as when a woman is not with child.

SECTION II.

Of the Difference between the Ancient and Modern Physicians, touching the Woman's contributing Seed to the Formation of the Child.

Our modern anatomists and physicians are of different sentiments from the ancients touching the woman's contributing of seed for the formation of the child, as well as the man; the ancients strongly affirming it, but our modern authors being generally of another judgment. I will not make myself a party in this controversy, but set down impartially, yet briefly, the arguments on each side, and leave the judicious reader to judge for himself.

Though it is apparent, say the ancients, that the seed of man is the principal efficient and beginning of action, motion, and generation, yet that the woman affords seed, and contributes to the procreation of the child, is evident from hence, that the women have seminal vessels, which had been given her in vain if she wanted seminal excrescence; but since nature forms nothing in vain, it must be granted they were made for the use of seed and procreation, and fixed in their proper places, to operate and contribute virtue and efficacy to the seed; and this, say they, is further proved from hence, that if women at years of maturity use not copulation to eject their seed, they often fall into strange diseases, as appears by young women and virgins: and also it appears that the women are never better pleased than when they are often satisfied this way, which argues that the pleasure and delight, say they, is double in women to what it is in men; for as the delight of men in copulation consists chiefly in the emission of the seed, so women are delighted both in the emission of their own and the reception of the man's.

But against all this, our modern authors affirm, that the ancients are very erroneous, inasmuch as the testicles in women do not afford seed, but are two eggs, like those of fowls and other creatures; neither have they any such offices as in men, but are indeed an ovarium, or recepticle for eggs, wherein these eggs are nourished by the sanguinary vessels dispersed through them; and from thence one or more, as they have fecundated by the man's seed, are conveyed into the womb by the ovaducts. And the truth of this, say they, is so plain, that if you boil them, their liquor will have the same taste, colour, and consistency, with the taste of birds' eggs. And if it be objected, that they have no shell, the answer is easy: for the eggs of fowls, while they are in the ovary, nay, after they are fallen snto the uterus, have no shell; and though they have one when they are laid, yet is no more than a fence which nature has provided for them against outward injuries, they being hatched without the body; but those of women being hatched within the body have no need of any other fence than the womb to secure them.

They also further say, there are in the generation of the fœtus, or young ones, two principles, *active* and *passive*: the *active* is the man's seed elaborated in the testicles, out of the arterial blood and animal spirit; the *passive* principle is the ovum, or egg, impregnated by the man's seed: for to say that women have true seed, say they, is erroneous. But the manner of conception is this: the most spirituous part of man's seed, in the act of copulation, reaching up to the ovarum or testicles of the woman (which contain divers eggs, sometimes more, sometimes fewer,) impregnates one of them; which, being conveyed by the ovaduct to the bottom of the womb, presently begins to swell bigger and bigger, and drinks in the moisture that is plentifully sent thither, after the same manner that the seeds in the ground suck in the fertile moisture thereof to make them sprout.

But, notwithstanding what is here urged by our modern anatomists, there are some late writers of the opinion of the ancients, viz. that women both have, and emit seed in the act of copulation; and even women themselves take ill to be thought merely passive in that act wherein they make such vigorous exertion, and positively affirm, that they are sensible of the emission of their seed in that action, and that in it a great part of the delight which they take in that action consists. I shall not, therefore, go about to take away any of their happiness from them, but leave them in possession of their imaginary felicity.

Having thus laid the foundation of this work, I will now proceed to speak of conception, and of those things that are necessary to be observed by women from the time of their conception to the time of their delivery.

K

CHAPTER II.

OF CONCEPTION; WHAT IT IS; HOW WOMEN ARE TO ORDER THEMSELVES AFTER CONCEPTION.

SECTION I.

What Conception is, and the Qualifications requisite thereto.

CONCEPTION is nothing else but an action of the womb, by which the prolific seed is received and retained, that an infant may be engendered and formed out of it. There are two sorts of conception: the one according to nature, which is followed by the generation of the infant in the womb; the other false, and wholly against nature, in which the seed changes into water, and produces only false conceptions, moles, or other strange matter. Now, there are three things particularly necessary in order to a true conception, so that generation may follow, viz. diversity of sex, congression, and emission of seed. Without diversity of sex there can be no conception; for, though some will have a women to be an animal that can engender of herself, it is a great mistake; there can be no conception without a man to discharge his seed into her womb. What they alledge of pullets laying eggs without a cock's treading them is nothing to the purpose; for those eggs, should they be set under a hen, will never become chickens, because they never received any prolific virtue from the male, which is absolutely necessary to this purpose, and is sufficient to convince us, that diversity of sex is necessary even to those animals, as well as to the generation of man. But diversity of sex, though it be necessary to conception, yet it will not do alone; there must also be a congression of those different sexes; for diversity of sex would profit little, if copulation did not follow. I confess I have heard of some subtle women, who, to cover their sin and shame, have endeavoured to persuade some peasants that they were never touched by man to get them with child; and that one, in particular, pretended to conceive by going into a bath where a man had washed himself a little before, and spent his seed in it, which was drawn and sucked into her womb, as she pretended. But such stories as these are only for those who know no better. Now, that these different sexes should be obliged to come to the touch, which we call copulation, or coition, besides the natural desire of begetting their like, which stirs up men and women to it, the parts appointed for generation are endowed by nature with a delightful and mutual itch, which begets in them a desire to the action; without which, it would not be very easy for a man, born for the contemplation of divine mysteries, to join himself by the way of coition, to a woman, in regard of the uncleanness of the part and of the action. And on the other side, if women did but think of those pains and inconveniences to which they are subject by their great bellies, and those hazards of life itself, besides the unavoidable pains that attend their delivery, it is reasonable to believe they would be affrighted from it. But neither sex makes these reflections till after the action is over, considering nothing beforehand but the pleasure of enjoyment; so that it is from this voluptuous itch that nature obliges both sexes to this congregation. Upon which the third thing followeth of course, viz. the emission of seed into the womb in the act of copulation. For the woman having received this prolific seed into her womb, and retained it there, the womb thereupon becomes depressed, and embraces the seed so closely, that being closed, the point of a needle cannot enter it without violence. And now the woman may be said to have conceived, having reduced by her heat from power into action the several faculties which are in the seed contained, making use of the spirits with which the seed abounds, and which are the instruments which begin to trace out the first lineaments of all the parts, and which afterwards, by making use of the menstruous blood flowing to it, give it, in time, growth and final perfection. And thus much shall suffice to explain what conception is. I shall now proceed to show,

SECTION II.

How a Woman ought to order herself after Conception.

My design in this treatise being brevity, I shall bring forward a little of what the learned have said of the causes of twins, and whether there be any such thing as superfoetations, or a second conception, in a woman, (which is yet common enough) when I come to show you how the midwife ought to proceed in the delivery of these women that are pregnant with them. But, having already spoke of conception, I think it now necessary to show how such as have conceived ought to order themselves during their pregnancy, that they may avoid those inconveniences which often endanger the life of the child, and many times their own.

A woman, after her conception, during the time of her being with child, ought to be looked on as indisposed or sick, though in good health; for child-bearing is a kind of one month's sickness, being all that time in expectation of many inconveniences which such a condition usually causes to those that are not well governed during that time; and therefore ought to resemble a good pilot, who, when sailing on a rough sea, and full of rocks, avoids and shuns the danger, if he steers with prudence; but if not, it is a thousand to one but he suffers shipwreck. In like manner, a woman with child is often in danger of miscarrying and losing her life, if she is not very careful to prevent those accidents to which she is subject all the time of her pregnancy; all which time her care must be double, first of herself, and secondly of the child she goes with; for otherwise, a single error may produce a double mischief; for, if she receives any prejudice, her child also suffers with her. Let a woman, therefore, after conception, observe a good diet, suitable to her temperament, custom, condition, and quality: and if she can, let the air where she ordinarily dwells be clear and well-tempered, free from extremes either of heat or cold; for being too hot it dissipateth the spirits too much, and causeth many weaknesses; and by being too cold and foggy, it may bring down rheums and distillations on the lungs, and so cause her to cough, which by its impetuous motion, forcing downwards, may make her miscarry. She ought also to avoid all nauseous and ill smells; for sometimes the stench of a candle, not well put out, may cause her to come before her time; and I have known the smell of charcoal to have the same effect. Let her also avoid of smelling of rue, mint, pennyroyal, castor, brimstone, &c.

But, with respect to their diet, women with child have generally so great loathings, and so many different longings, that it is very difficult to prescribe an exact diet for them. Only this I think advisable, that they may use those meats and drinks which are to them most desirable, though perhaps not in themselves so wholesome as some others, and it may be, not so pleasant; but this liberty must be made use of with this caution, that what she so desires be not in itself unwholesome; and also, that in every thing she take care of excess.

But, if a child-bearing woman finds herself not troubled with such longings as we have spoken of, let her take simple food, and in such quantity as may be sufficient for herself and the child, which her appetite may in a great measure regulate; for it is alike hurtful to her to fast too long, or to eat too much: and, therefore, rather let her eat a little and often: especially let her avoid eating too much at night; because the stomach being too much filled compresseth the diaphragms, and thereby causes difficulty of breathing. Let her meat be easy of digestion, such as the tenderest parts of beef, mutton, veal, sows, pullets, capons, pigeons, and patridges, either boiled or roasted, as she likes best; new laid eggs are also very good for her; and let her put into her broths those herbs that purify it, as sorrel, lettuce, succory, and burrage: for they will purge and purify the blood. Let her avoid whatsoever is hot seasoned, especially pies and baked meats, which, being of hot digestion, overcharge the stomach. If she desires fish, let it be fresh, and such as is taken out of rivers and running streams. Let her eat quinces or marmalade, to strengthen her child; for which purpose sweet almonds, honey, sweet apples, and full ripe grapes, are also good. Let her abstain from all sharp, sour, bitter, and salt things; and all things that tend to provoke the terms—such as garlic, onions, olives, mustard, fennel, pepper, and all spices except cinnamon, which in the last three months is good for her. If at first her diet be sparing, as she increases in bigness let her diet be increased: for she ought to consider she has a child as well as herself to nourish. Let her be moderate in her drinking; and if she drinks wine, let it be rather claret than white, (which will breed good blood, help the digestion, and comfort the stomach, which is always weakly during her pregnancy,) but white wine being diuretic, or that which provokes urine, ought to be avoided. Let her have a care of too much exercise; and let her avoid dancing, riding in a coach, or whatever else puts the body into violent motion, especially in her first month. But to be more particular, I shall here set down rules proper for every month for child bearing women to order herself, and from the time she first conceived to the time of her delivery.

Rules for the First Two Months

As soon as a woman knows (or has reason to believe) she hath conceived she ought to abstain from all violent motions and exercise; whether she walks on foot, or rides on horseback, or in a coach, it ought to be very gently. Let her also abstain from every venery (to which, after conception, she has usually no great inclination,) lest there be a mole or superfœtation; which is the adding of one embryo to another. Let her beware she lift not her arms too high, nor carry great burdens, nor repose herself on hard and uneasy seats. Let her use moderately good juicy meat, and of easy digestion;

and let her wine be neither too strong nor too sharp, but a little mingled with water; or if she be very abstemious, she may use water wherein cinnamon is boiled. Let her avoid fastings, thirst, watching, mourning, sadness, anger, and all other perturbations of the mind. Let none present any strange or unwholesome thing to her, nor so much as name it, lest she should desire it, and not be able to get it, and so either cause her to miscarry, or the child to have some deformity on that account. Let her belly be kept loose with prunes, raisins, or manna, in her broth; and let her use the following electuary, to strengthen the womb and the child:

"Take conserve of burrage, buglos, and red roses, each two ounces; of balm an ounce; citron peel and shreds, mirobolans candied, each an ounce; extract of wood aloes, a scruple; pearl prepared, half a dram; red coral, ivory, each a dram; precious stones, each a scruple; candied nutmegs, two drams: and with syrup of apples and quinces make an electuary."

Let her observe the following Rules.

"Take pearls prepared, a dram; red coral prepared and ivory, each half a dram; precious stones, each a scruple; yellow citron peels, mace, cinnamon, cloves, each half a dram; saffron, a scruple; wood aloes, half a scruple; ambergris, six drams; and with six ounces of sugar dissolved in rose-water, make rolls." Let her also apply strengtheners to the navel, of nutmegs, mace, mastich, made up in bags, or a toast dipt in malmsey, sprinkled with powder of mint. If she happens to desire clay, chalk, or coals (as many women with child do,) give her beans boiled with sugar; and if she happens to long for any thing which she cannot obtain, let her presently drink a large draught of pure cold water.

Rules for the Third Month.

In his month and the next, be sure to keep from bleeding; for though it may be safe and proper at other times, it will not be so to the end of the fourth month: and yet if too much blood abound, or some incident disease happen, which requires evacuation, you may use a cupping-glass, with sacrification, and a little blood may be drawn from the shoulders and arms, especially if she has been accustomed to bleed. Let her also take care of lacing herself too straitly, but give herself more liberty than she used to do; for, inclosing her belly in too straight a mould, she hinders the infant from taking its free growth, and often makes it come before its time.

Rules for the Fourth Month.

In this month you ought to keep the childbearing woman from bleeding, unless in extraordinary cases; but when this month is past, bloodletting and physic may be permitted, if it be gentle and mild; and perhaps it may be necessary to prevent abortion. In this month she may purge in an acute disease; but purging may be only used from the beginning of this month to the end of the sixth: but let her take care that in purging she use no vehement medicine, nor any bitter, as aloes, which is disagreeable and hurtful to the child, and opens the mouth of the vessels; neither let her use coloquintida, scammony, nor turbith: she may use cassia, manna, rhubarb, agaric, and senna: but dyacidodium purgans is best, with a little of the electuary of the juice of roses.

Rules for the Fifth, Sixth, and Seventh Months.

In these months childbearing women are troubled with coughs, heartbeating, fainting, watching, pains in the loins and hips, and bleeding. The cough is from a sharp vapour that comes to the jaws and rough artery from the terms, or the thin part of that blood gotten into the veins of the breast; or falling from the head to the breast; this endangers abortion, and strength fails from watching; therefore purge the humours that fall to the breast with rhubarb and agaric, and strengthen the head as in a catarrh, and give sweet lenitives, as in a cough. Palpatation and fainting arise from vapours that go to it by the arteries, or from blood that aboundeth, and cannot get out at the womb, but ascends, and oppresseth the heart; and in this case cordials should be used both inwardly and outwardly. Watching is from sharp dry vapours that trouble the animal spirits, and in this case use frictions, and let the woman wash her feet at bed-time, and let her take syrup of poppies, dried roses, emulsions of sweet almonds, and white poppy seed. If she be troubled with pains in her loins and hips, as in these months she is subject to be from the weight of her child, who is now grown big and heavy, and so stretcheth the ligaments of the womb, and parts adjacent, let her hold it up with swathing bands about her neck. About this time also the woman often happens to have a flux of blood; either at the nose, womb, or hemorrhoids, from plenty of blood, or from the weakness of the child that takes it not in in; or else from evil humour in the blood, that stirs up nature to send it forth. And sometimes it happens that the vessels of the womb may be broken, either by some violent motion, fall, cough, or trouble of mind, (for any of these will work that effect;) and this is so dangerous, that in such a case the child cannot be well; but if it be from blood only, the danger is less, provided it flows by the veins of the neck of the womb; for then it prevents plethory, and takes not away the nourishment of the child; but if it proceeds from the weakness of the child, that draws it not in, abortion of the child often follows, or hard travail, or else she goes beyond her time. But if it flows by the inward veins of the womb, there is more danger by the openness of the womb, if it come from evil blood; the danger is alike from cacochimi, which is like to fall upon both. If it arises from plethory, open a vein, but with very great caution, and use astringents, of which the following will do well:— take pearls prepared, a scruple; red coral, two scruples; mace, nutmegs, each a dram; cinnamon, half a dram; make a powder, or, with sugar, rolls. Or give this powder in broth; "Take red coral, a dram; half a dram precious stones: red sander, half a dram: sealed earth, tormentil roots, each two scruples, with sugar of roses, and manus Christi: with pearl, five drams: make a powder. You may also strengthen the child at the navel: and if there be a cachochimy, alter the humours: and if you may do it safely, evacuate: you may likewise use amulets in her hands and about her neck. In a flux of hemorrhoids, wear off the pain; and let her drink hot wine with a toasted nutmeg. In these months the belly is also subject to be bound; but if it be without any apparent disease, the broth of a chicken, or veal sodden with oil, or with the decoction of mallows, or marshmallows, mercury, and linseed, put up in a clyster, will not be amiss, but in less quantity than is given in other cases: viz. of the decoction five ounces, of common oil three ounces, of sugar two ounces, of cassia fistula one ounce. But if she will not take a clyster, one or two yolks of new laid eggs, or a little peas' pottage warm, with a little salt and sugar, supped a little before meat, will be very convenient. But if her belly shall be distended and stretched out with wind, a little fennel seed and anniseed reduced into powder, and mingled with honey and sugar, made after the manner of an electuary, will do very well. Also, if the thighs and feet swell, let them be anointed with exphrodinum (which is a liquid medicine made with vinegar and rose-water,) mingled with salt.

Rules for the Eighth Month.

The eighth is commonly the most dangerous, therefore the greatest care and caution ought to be used; the diet better in quality but not more, nor indeed so much in quantity as before; but as she must abate her diet, so she must increase her exercise: and because then women with child, by reason that sharp humours alter the belly, are accustomed to weaken their spirits and strength, they may well take before meat an electuary of diarrhoden or aromaticum rosatum, or diamagarton; and sometimes they may lick a little honey: as they will loathe and nauseate their meat, they may take green ginger candied with sugar, or the rinds of citron and oranges candied; and let them often use honey for the strengthening of the infant. When she is not far from her labour, let her eat every day seven roasted figs before meat, and sometimes let her lick a little honey. But let her beware of salt and powdered meat, for it is neither good for her nor the child.

Rules for the Ninth Month.

In the ninth month let her have a care of lifting any great weight; but let her move a little more, to dilate the parts and stir up natural heat. Let her take heed of stooping, and neither sit too much, nor lie on her sides; neither ought she to bend herself much, lest the child be unfolded in the umbilical ligament, by which means it often perisheth. Let her walk and stir often, and let her exercise be rather to go upwards than downwards. Let her diet, now especially, be light and easy of digestion; and damask prunes with sugar, or figs with raisins, before meat; as also the yolks of eggs, flesh and broth of chicken, birds, partridges, and pheasants; astringent and roasted meats, with rice, hard eggs, millet and such like other things are proper. Baths of sweet water, with emollient herbs, ought to be used by her this month with some intermission; and after the baths, let her belly be anointed with oil of roses and violets; but for her privy parts it is better to anoint them with the fat of hens, geese, or ducks, or with oil of lilies; and the decoction of linseed and fenugreek, boiled with oil of linseed and marshmallows, or with the following liniment:

"Take of mallows and marshmallows, cut and shred, of each an ounce; of linseed one ounce; let them be boiled from twenty ounces of water to ten; then let her take three ounces of the boiled broth; of oil of almonds and oil of flower-de-luce, of each one ounce; of deer's suet three ounces." Let her bathe with this, and anoint herself with it warm.

If for fourteen days before the birth she do every morning and evening bathe and moisten her belly with muscadine and lavender water, the child will be much strengthened thereby. And if every day she eat toasted bread, it will hinder any thing from growing to the child. Her privy parts may be gently stroked down with this fomentation.

"Take three ounces of linseed, and one handful each of mallows and marshmallows sliced, then let them be put in a bag and immediately boiled." Let the woman with child every morning and evening take the vapour of this decoction in a hollow stool, taking great heed that no wind or air come to her in-parts, and then let her wipe the part so anointed with a linen cloth, and she may anoint the belly and groins as at first.

When she is come so near her time as to be within ten or fourteen days thereof, if she begins to feel any more than ordinary pain, let her use every day the following:—"Take mallows and marshmallows, of each one handful; camomile, hard mercury, maiden-hair, of each half a handful; of linseed, four ounces; let them be boiled in such a sufficient quantity of water as to make a bath therewith." But let her not sit too hot upon the seat, nor higher than a little above her navel: nor let her sit on it longer than about half an hour, lest her strength languish and decay; for it is better to use it often than to stay too long in it.

And thus have I shown how a child bearing woman ought to govern herself each month during her pregnancy. How she must order herself at her delivery, shall be shown in another chapter, after I have first shown the intended midwife how the child is first formed in the womb, and the manner of its decumbiture there.

CHAPTER III.

Of the Parts proper to a Child in the Womb. How it is formed there, and the manner of its Situation therein.

IN the last chapter I treated of conception, showing what it was, how accomplished, its signs, and how she who has conceived ought to order herself during the time of her pregnancy. Now before I come to speak of her delivery, it is necessary that the midwife be first made acquainted with the parts proper to a child in the womb: and also, that she be shown how it is formed: and the manner of its situation and decumbiture there: which are so necessary to her, that without the knowledge thereof no one can tell how to deliver a woman as she ought. This, therefore, shall be the work of this chapter. I shall begin with the first of these.

SECTION I.

Of the Parts proper to a Child in the Womb.

In this section I must first tell you what I mean by the parts proper to the child in the womb; and they are only those that either help or nourish it, whilst it is lodged in that dark repository of nature, and that help to clothe and defend it there, and are cast away, as of no more use, after it is born; and these are two, viz. the umbilicurs, or navel vessels, and the secundinum. By the first it is nourished, and by the second clothed and defended from wrong. Of each of these I shall speak distinctly: and, first,

Of the Umbilicurs, or Navel Vessels.

These are four in number, viz. one vein, two arteries and the vessel which is called the urachos.

1. The vein is that by which the infant is nourished, from the time of its conception till the time of its delivery; till, being brought into the light of this world, it has the same way of concocting its food that we have. This vein ariseth from the liver of the child, and is divided into two parts when it hath passed the navel; and these two are again divided and subdivided, the branches being upheld by the skin called *chorion* (of which I shall speak by and by,) and are joined to the veins of the mother's womb, from whence they have their blood for the nourishment of the child.

2. The arteries are two on each side, which proceed from the back branches of the great artery of the mother; and the vital blood is carried by those to the child, being ready concocted by the mother.

3. A nervous or sinewy production is led from the bottom of the bladder of the infant to the navel, and this is called *urachos*; and its use is to convey the urine of the infant from the bladder to the alantois. Anatomists do very much vary in their opinions concerning this: some denying any such thing to be in the delivery of women: and others on the contrary, affirming it: but experience has testified there is such a thing; for Bartholomew Carbrolius, the ordinary doctor of anatomy to the College of Physicians at Montpelier, in France, records the history of a maid, whose water, being a long time stopped, at last issued out through her navel. And Johannes Fernelius speaks of the same thing that happened to a man of thirty years of age, who, having a stoppage at the

neck of the bladder, his urine issued out of his navel many months together, and that without any prejudice at all to his health; which he ascribes to the ill lying of his navel, whereby the urachos was not well dried. And Volchier Coitas quotes such another instance in a maid of 34 years of age, at Nuremburg, in Germany. These instances, though they happen but seldom, are very sufficient to prove that there is such a thing as an urachos in men.

These four vessels before-mentioned, viz. one vein, two arteries, and the urachos, do join near to the navel, and are united by a skin, which they have from the chorion, and so become like a gut or rope, and are altogether void of sense, and this is that which women call the navel-string. The vessels are thus joined together, that so they may neither be broken, severed, nor entangled: and when the infant is born, are of no use, save only to make up the ligament which stops the hole of the navel, and some other physical use, &c.

Of the Secundine, or After-Birth.

Setting aside the name given to this by the Greeks and Latins, it is called in English by the name of secundine, after-birth, or after-burden; which are held to be four in number.

1. The *first* is called placentia, because it resembles the form of a cake, and is knit both to the navel and chorion, and makes up the greatest part of the secundine, or after birth. The flesh of it is like that of the milt, or spleen, soft, red, and tending something to blackness, and hath many small veins and arteries in it; and certainly the chief use of it is, for containing the child in the womb.

2. The *second* is the chorion. This skin, and that called the amonis, involve the child round, both above and underneath, and on both sides, which the alantois doth not. This skin is that which is most commonly called the secundine, as it is thick and white, garnished with many small veins and arteries, ending in the placentia before named, being very light and slippery. Its use is not only to cover the child round about, but also to receive and safely bind up the roots of the veins and arteries or navel vessels before described.

3. The *third* thing which makes up the secundine is the alantois, of which there is a great dispute amongst anatomists. Some say, there is such a thing; and others that there is not. Those that will have it to be a membrane, say it is white, soft, and exceeding thin, and just under the placentia, where it is knit to the urachos, from whence it receives the urine; and its office is to keep it separate from the sweat,

that the saltness of it may not offend the tender skin of the child.

4. The *fourth* and last covering of the child, is called amnios; and it is white, soft, and transparent, being nourished by some very small veins and arteries. Its use is not only to enwrap the child, but also to retain the sweat of the child.

Having thus described the parts proper to a child in the womb, I will next proceed to speak of the formation of the child therein, as soon as I have explained the hard terms of this section, that those for whose help this is designed, may understand what they read. A *vein* is that which receives blood from the liver, and distributes it in several branches to all parts of the body. *Arteries* proceed from the heart, are in a continual motion, and by their continual motion quicken the body. *Nerve* is the same with *sinew*, and is that by which the brain adds sense and motion to the body. *Placentia* properly signifies *a sugar cake;* but in this section it is used to signify a spungy piece of flesh, resembling a cake, full of veins and arteries, and is made to receive the mother's blood appointed for the infant's nourishment in the womb. The *chorion* is the outward skin which compasseth the child in the womb. The *amnios* is the inner skin which compasseth the child in the womb. The *alantois* is the skin that holds the urine of the child during the time that it abides in the womb. The *urachos* is the vessel that conveys the urine from the child in the womb to the *alantois*. I now proceed to

SECTION II.

Of the Formation of the Child in the Womb.

To speak of the formation of the child in the womb, we must begin where nature begins; and that is at the act of coition, in which the womb having received the generative seed (without which there can be no conception,) the womb immediately shuts up itself so close that the point of a needle cannot enter the inward orifice; and this it does partly to hinder the issuing out of the seed again, and partly to cherish it by an inbred heat, the better to provoke it to action which is one reason why women's bellies are so lank at their first conception. The woman having thus conceived, the first thing which is operative in the conception is the spirit, whereof the seed is full, which nature quickening by the heat of the womb, stirs up to action. This seed consists of very different parts, of which some are more, and some are less

L

pure. The internal spirits, therefore, separate the parts that are less pure, which are thick, cold, and clammy, from those that are more pure and noble. The less pure are cast to the outsides, and with these the seed is circled round, and the membranes made, in which that seed which is the most pure is wrapped round, and kept close together, that it may be defended from cold and other accidents, and operate the better.

The first thing that is formed is the amnios; the next the chorion; and they enwrap the seed round like a curtain. Soon after this (for the seed thus shut up in the woman lies not idle) the navel vein is bred, which pierceth those skins, being yet very tender, and carries a drop of blood from the veins of the mother's womb to the seed, from which the vena cava, or chief vein, proceeds; from which all the rest of the veins which nourish the body, spring; and now the seed hath something to no nourish it, whilst it performs the rest of nature's work, and also blood administered to every part of it, to form flesh.

This vein being formed, the navel arteries are soon after formed; then the great artery, of which all others are but branches; and then the heart: for the liver furnisheth the arteries with blood to form the heart: the arteries being made of seed, but the heart and the flesh of blood. After this the brain is formed, and then the nerves to give sense and motion to the infant. Afterwards the bones and flesh are formed; and of the bones, first the vertebræ or chin bones, and then the skull, &c.

As to the time in which this curious part of nature's workmanship is formed, having already in Chapter II. of the former part of this work. spoken at large upon this point, and also of the nourishment of the child in the womb, I shall here only refer the reader thereto, and proceed to show the manner in which the child lies in the womb.

SECTION III.

Of the Manner of the Child's lying in the Womb.

This is a thing so essential for a midwife to know, that she can be no midwife who is ignorant of it: and yet even about this authors extremely differ; for there are not two in ten that agree what is the form that the child lies in the womb, or in what fashion it lies there; and yet this may arise in a great measure from the different figures that the child is found in, according to the different times of the woman's pregnancy; for near the time of its deliverance out of those winding chambers of nature, it oftentimes changes the form in which it lay before for another.

I will now show the several situations of the child in the mother's womb, according to the different times of pregnancy, by which those that are contrary to nature, and are the chief cause of all ill labours, will be the more easily conceived by the understanding midwife. It ought, therefore, in the first place, to be observed, that the infant, as well male as female, is generally situated in the midst of the womb; for though sometimes, to appearance, a woman's belly seems higher on one side than another, yet it is so with respect to her belly only, and not to her womb, in the midst of which it is always placed.

But, in the second place, a woman's great belly makes different figures, according to the different times of pregnancy; for, when she is young with child, the embryo is always found of a round figure, a little oblong, having the spine moderately turned inwards, the thighs folded, and a little raised, to which the legs are so raised, that the heels touch the buttocks; the arms are bending, and the hands placed upon the knees towards which the head is inclining forwards, so that the chin toucheth the breast; in which posture it resembles one sitting to ease nature, and stooping down with the head to see what comes from him. The spine of its back is at that time placed towards the mother's, the head uppermost, the face forwards, and the feet downwards; and, proportionably to its growth, it extends its members by little and little, which were exactly folded in the first month. In this posture it usually keeps till the seventh or eighth month; and then, by a natural propensity and disposition of the upper part of the body, the head is turned downwards toward the inward orifice of the womb, tumbling as it were over its head, so that then the feet are uppermost, and the face towards the mother's great gut: and this turning of the infant in this manner, with its head downwards, towards the latter end of a woman's reckoning, is so ordered by nature, that it may thereby be the better disposed for its passage into the world at the time of its mother's labour, which is not then far off (and indeed some children turn not at all, until the very time of birth) for in this posture all its joints are most easily extended in coming forth; for, by this means the arms and legs cannot hinder its birth, because they cannot be bended against the inward orifice of the womb; and the rest of the body being very supple, passeth without any difficulty after the head, which is hard and big, being past the birth. It is true, there are divers children that lie in the womb in another posture, and come to birth with their feet downwards, especially if there be twins; for then by the different motions they do so disturb one another, that they seldom come both in the same posture at the time of labour, but one will come with the head, and another with the feet, or perhaps lie across; and sometimes neither of them will come right. But however the child may be situated in the womb, or in whatever posture it presents itself at the time of birth, if it be not with its head forwards, as I have before described, it is always against nature, and the delivery will occasion the mother more pain and danger, and require greater care and skill from the midwife, than when the labour is more natural.

CHAPTER IV.

A Guide for Women in Travail, showing what is to be done, when they fall in Labour, in order to their Delivery.

THE end of all we have been treating of is, the bringing forth a child into the world with safety both to the mother and the infant, as the whole time of a woman's pregnancy may very well be termed a kind of labour; for, from the time of her conception to the time of her delivery, she labours under many difficulties, is subject to many distempers, and in continual danger, from one effect or another, till the time of birth comes, and when that comes the greatest labour comes with it, insomuch, that her labours are forgotten, and that only is called the time of her labour; and to deliver her safely is the principal business of the midwife; and to assist her therein shall be the chief design of this chapter. The time of the child's being ready for its birth, when nature endeavours to cast it forth, is that which is properly the time of a woman's labour; nature then labouring to be eased of its burden. And since many child-bearing women (especially the first child) are often mistaken in their reckoning, and so, when they draw near their time, take every pain they meet with for their labour, which often proves prejudicial and troublesome to them, when it is not so; I will, in the first section of this chapter, set down some signs, by which a woman may know when the true time of her labour is come.

SECTION I.

The Signs of the true Time of a Woman's Labour.

When women with child, especially of their first, perceive any extraordinary pains in their belly, they immediately send for their midwife, as taking it for labour; and then, if the midwife be not a skilful and experienced women to know the time of labour, but takes it for granted without further inquiry, (for some such there are,) and so goes about to put her into labour before nature is prepared for it, she may endanger the lives of both mother and child, by breaking the amnios and chorion. These pains, which are often mistaken for labour, are removed by warm cloths laid to the belly, and the application of a clyster or two, by which those pains which precede a true labour are rather furthered than hindered. There are also other pains incident to a woman in that condition from a flux of the belly, which are easily known by the frequent stools that follow them.

The signs, therefore, of labour, some few days before, are that the woman's belly, which before lay high, sinks down, and hinders her from walking so easily as she used to do; also there flows from the womb slimy humours, which nature has appointed to moisten and smooth the passage, that its inward orifice may be the more easily dilated when there is occasion: which, beginning to open at that time, suffers that slime to flow away, which proceeds from the glandules, called *prostata*. These are signs preceding the labour; but when she is presently falling into labour, the signs are, great pains about he region of the reins and loins, which, coming and retreating by intervals, are answered in the bottom of the belly by congruous throws, and sometimes the face is red and inflamed, the blood being much heated by the endeavours a woman makes to bring forth her child; and likewise, because during these strong throws her respiration is intercepted which causes the blood to have recourse to her face; also her privy parts are swelled by the infant's head lying in the birth, which, by often thrusting, causes those parts to descend outwards. She is much subject to vomiting, which is a sign of good labour and speedy delivery, though by ignorant women thought otherwise; for good pains are thereby excited and redoubled; which vomiting is excited by the sympathy there is between the womb and the stomach. Also, when the birth is near, women are troubled with trembling in the thighs and legs, not with cold like the beginning of an ague fit, but with the heat of the whole body: though it must be granted, this does not happen always. Also, if the humours which then flow from the womb are discoloured with the blood, which the midwives call *shows*, it is an infallible mark of the birth being near. And if then the midwife puts up her fingers into the neck of the womb, she will find the inner orifice dilated; at the opening of which, the membranes of the infant, containing the water, present themselves, and are strongly forced downwards with each pain she hath; at which time one may perceive them sometimes to resist, and then again press forward the finger, being more or less hard and extended, according as the pains are stronger or weaker. These membranes, with the waters in them, when they are before the head of the child, which the midwives call *the gathering of the waters*, resemble to the touch of the finger those eggs which have no shell, but are covered only by a simple membrane. After this, the pains still redoubling, the membranes are broken by a strong impulsion of the waters, which flow away, and then the head of the infant is presently felt naked, and presents itself at the inward orifice of her womb. When these waters come thus away, then the midwife may be assured the birth is very near, this being the most certain sign that can be; for the *amnios alantois*, which contained those waters being broken by the pressing forward of the birth, the child is no better able to subsist long in the womb afterwards, than a naked man in a heap of snow.

Now, these waters, if the child comes presently after them, facilitate the labour, by making the passage slippery; and, therefore, let no midwife (as some have foolishly done) endeavour to force away the water, for nature knows best when the true time of the birth is, and therefore retains the water till that time. But if by accident the water breaks away too long before the birth, then such things as will hasten it may be safely administered; and what these are, I shall show in another section.

SECTION II.

How a Woman ought to be ordered when the Time of her Labour is come

When it is known that the true time of her labour is come, by the signs laid down in the foregoing section, of which those that are most to be relied on are pains and strong throws in the belly, forcing downwards towards the womb, and a dilation of the inward orifice, may be perceived by touching it with the finger, and the gathering of the waters before the head of the child, and thrusting down of the membranes which contain them; through which, between the pains, one may in some manner with the finger discover the part which presents (as was said before,) especially if it be the head of the child, by its roundness and hardness; I say, if these things concur and are evident, the midwife may be sure it is the time of the woman's labour; and care must be taken to get all things that are necessary to comfort her in that time. And the better to help her, be sure to see she be not strait-laced; you may also give her one strong clyster or more, if there be occasion, provided it be none at the beginning, and before the child be too forward; for it will be difficult for her to receive them afterwards. The benefit accruing hereby will be, that they excite the gut to discharge itself of its excrements, that so, the rectum being emptied, there may be more space for the dilation of the passage: likewise to cause the pains to bear the more downward, through the endeavours she makes when she is at stool: and in the meantime, all other necessary things for her labour should be put in order, both for the mother and child. To this end some get a midwife's stool; but a pallet bed, girded, is much the best way, placed near the fire, if the season so require; which pallet ought to be so placed, that there may be easy access to it on every side, that the women may be more readily assisted as there is occasion.

If the woman abounds with blood, to bleed her a little may not be improper, for thereby she will both breathe the better and have her breasts more at liberty, and likewise more strength to bear down her pains; and this may be done without danger, because the child being about that time ready to be born, has no more need of the mother's blood for its nourishment: besides, this evacuation does many times prevent her having a fever after delivery, and if her strength permit, let her walk up and down her chamber: and that she may have strength so to do, it will be necessary to give her some good strengthening things, such as jelly broth, new laid eggs, or some spoonsful of burnt wine; and let her by all means hold out her pains, bearing them down as much as she can at the time they take her; and let the midwife from time to time touch the inward orifice with her finger, to know whether the waters are ready to break, and whether the birth will follow soon after. Let her also anoint the woman's privities with emollient oil, hogs' grease, and fresh butter, if she find they are hard to be dilated. Let the midwife likewise be all the while near the labouring woman, and diligently observe her gestures, complaints, and pains; for by this she may guess pretty well how her labour advanceth because when she changeth her ordinary groans into loud cries, it is a sign the child is very near the birth; for at that time her pains are greater and more frequent. Let the woman, likewise by intervals, rest herself on the bed, to regain her strength, but not too long, especially if she be little, short, and thick; for such women have always worse labour if they lie long on their beds in their travail. It is better, therefore that she walk about the chamber as much as she can, the women supporting her under the arms, if it be necessary: for by this means, the weight of the child causeth the inward orifice of the womb to dilate the sooner than in bed; and if her pains be stronger and more frequent, her labour will not be near so long.

Let not the labouring woman be concerned at those qualms and vomitings which perhaps she may find come upon her, for they will be much for her advantage in the issue, however uneasy she may be for the time, as they further her throes and pains by provoking downwards.

When the waters of the child are ready and gathered, (as may be perceived through the membranes to present themselves to the inward orifice) to the bigness of the whole dilation, the midwife ought to let them break of themselves, and not, like some hasty midwives, who being impatient of the woman's long labour, break them, intending thereby to hasten their business, when instead thereof they retard it, for, by the too hasty breaking of these waters (which nature designed to cause the infant to slide forth more easy) the passage remains dry, by which means the pains and throws of the labouring women are less efficacious to bring forth the infant than they would otherwise have been. It is therefore much the better way to let the waters break of themselves; after which the midwife may with ease feel the child by that part which presents, and thereby discern whether it comes right; that is with the head foremost, for that is the most proper and natural way of its birth. If the head comes right, she will find it round, big, hard, and equal; but if it be any other part, she will feel it unequal, rugged, and soft or hard, according to the nature of the part it is. And this being the true time when the woman ought to be delivered, if nature be not wanting to perform its office; therefore, when the midwife finds the birth thus coming forward, let her hasten to assist and deliver it, for it ordinarily happens soon after, if it be natural.

But if it happens, as sometimes it may, that the waters break away too long before the birth, in such a case those things that hasten nature may be safely administered. For which purpose make use of penny-royal, dittany, juniper-berries, red coral, betony, and feverfew, boiled in white wine, and give a draught of it; or it would be much better to take the juice of it when in its prime, which is in May, and having clarified it, make it into syrup, with double its weight of sugar, and keep it all the year, to use when occasion calls for it: mugwort, used in the same manner, is also good in this case; also a dram of cinnamon powder given inwardly, profits much in this case; and so does tansey, broiled, and applied to the privities; or an oil of it, so made and used, as you were taught before. The stone Ætites held to the privities is of extraordinary virtue, and instantly draws away both child and after-burden; but great care must be taken to remove it presently, or it will draw forth the womb and all; for such is the magnetic virtue of this stone, that both child and womb follow it as readily as iron doth the loadstone, or the loadstone the north star.

There are many other things that physicians affirm are good in this case; among which are, an ass's or horse's hoof hung near the privities; a piece of red coral hung near the said place. A loadstone helps very much, held in the woman's left hand; or the skin cut off a snake, girt about the middle, next the skin. These things are mentioned by Mizaldus; but setting those things aside, as not so certain, notwithstanding Mizaldus quotes them, the following prescriptions are very good to give speedy deliverance to women in travail.

1. A decoction of white wine made in savory, and drank.

2. Take wild tansey, or silver-weed, bruise it, and apply it to the woman's nostrils.

3. Take date-stones, and beat them to powder, and let her take half a dram of them in white wine at a time.

4. Take parsley, and bruise it, and press out the juice, and dip a linen cloth in it, and put it up so dipped into the mouth of the womb; it will presently cause the child to come away, though it be dead, and will bring away the after-burden.

Also, the juice of parsley is a thing of so great virtue (especially stone-parsley) that being drank by a woman with child it cleanseth not only the womb, but also the child in the womb, of all gross humours.

5. A scruple of castorum in powder, in any convenient liquor, is very good to be taken in such a case; and so also is two or three drops of spirit of castorum in any convenient liquor; also eight or nine drops of spirit of myrrh, given in any convenient liquor, gives speedy deliverance.

6. Give a woman in such a case another woman's milk to drink: it will cause speedy delivery, and almost without any pain.

7. The juice of leeks, being drank with warm water, highly operates to cause speedy delivery.

8. Take peony-seeds, and beat them into powder, and mix the powder with oil, with which oil anoint the loins and privities of the woman and child: it will give her deliverance very speedily, and with less pain than can be imagined.

9. Take a swallow's nest, and dissolve it in water, strain it and drink it warm; it gives delivery with great speed and much ease.

Note this also in general, that all things that move the terms, are good for making the delivery easy; such as myrrh, white amber in white wine, or lilly-water, two scruples or a dram: or cassia lignea, dittany, each a dram; cinnamon half a dram, saffron, a scruple; give a dram: or take borax mineral a dram, cassia lignea a scruple, saffron six grains, and give it in sack; or take cassia lignea a dram; dittany, amber, of each a dram; cinnamon, borax, of each a dram and a half; saffron a scruple; and give her half a dram; or give her some drops of oil of hazel in convenient liquor; or two or three drops of oil of cinnamon in vervain water. Some prepare the secundine thus: Take the navel-string and dry it in an oven, take two drams of the powder, cinnamon a dram, saffron half a scruple, with juice of savin make trochisks; give two drams; or wash the secundine in wine, and bake it in a pot; then wash it in endive water and wine; take half a dram of it: long pepper, galengal, of each half a dram; plantain and endive seed, of each a dram and a half; lavender seed four scruples; make a powder; or take laudanum two drams; storax, calamite, benzoin, of each half a dram; musk, ambergreise, each six grains; make a powder, or trochisks for a fume. Or use pessaries to provoke the birth: take galbanum dissolved in vinegar, an ounce; myrrh two drams; saffron a dram; with oil of orris make a pessary.

An Ointment for the Navel.

Take oil of keir two ounces, juice of savine an ounce, of leeks and mercury each half an ounce; boil them to the consumption of the juice; and galbanum dissolved in vinegar half an ounce, myrrh two drams, storax liquid a dram: round bitwort sowbread, cinnamon, saffron a dram; with wax make an ointment, and apply it.

If the birth be retarded through the weakness of the mother, refresh her by applying wine and soap to the nose; confect, alkermes diamarg

These things may be applied to help nature in the delivery, when the child comes to the birth the right way, and yet the birth be retarded; but if she finds the child comes the wrong way, and is not able to deliver the woman as she ought to be, by helping nature and saving both mother and child (for it is not enough to lay a woman, if it might be done any other way with more safety and ease, and less hazard both to woman and child,) then let her send speedily for better and more able help; and not, as I once knew a midwife do, who, when a woman she was to deliver had hard labour, rather than a man-midwife should be sent for, undertook to deliver the woman herself (though told it was a man's business,) and in her attempting it brought away the child, but left the head of the infant in the mother's womb: and had not a man-midwife been presently sent for, the mother had lost her life as well as the child: such persons may rather be termed butchers than midwives. But supposing the woman's labour to be natural, I will next show what the midwife ought to do, in order to her delivery.

CHAPTER V.

Of Natural Labour; what it is, and what the Midwife is to do in such a Labour.

SECTION I. *What Natural Labour is.*

There are four things which denominate a woman's natural labour: the first is, that it be at the full time; for, if a woman comes before her time, it cannot properly be termed natural labour; neither will it be so easy as if she had completed her nine months. The second thing is, that it be speedy, and without an ill accident: for, when the time of the birth is come, nature is not dilatory in the bringing of it forth without some ill accident intervene, which renders it unnatural. The third is, that the child be alive; for all will grant, that the being delivered of a dead child is very unnatural. The fourth thing requisite to a natural birth is, that the child come right: for if the position of the child in the womb be contrary to what is natural, the event will prove it so, by making that which should be a time of life the death both of the mother and the child.

Having thus told you what I mean by natural labour, I shall next show how the midwife is to proceed therein, in order to the woman's delivery. When all the foregoing requisites concur, and after the waters be broke of themselves, let the labouring woman be conducted to a pallet bed, provided near the fire for that purpose, as has already been said, and let there rather be a quilt laid upon the pallet bedstead than a feather bed, having thereon linen, and cloths in many folds, with such other things as are necessary, and that may be changed according to the exigency requiring it, so that the woman may not be incommoded with the blood, waters, and other filth which are avoided in labour. The bed ought so to be ordered, that the woman, being ready to be delivered, should lie on her back upon it, having her body in a convenient posture; that is, her head and breast a little raised, so that she be between lying and sitting; for being so placed, she is best capable of breathing, and likewise will have more strength to bear her pains than if she lay otherwise, or sunk down in her bed. Being so placed, she must spread her thighs abroad, folding her legs a little towards her buttocks, somewhat raised by a small pillow underneath, to the end her rump should have more liberty to retire back; and let her feet be stayed against some firm thing: besides this, let her take hold of some of the good women attending her with her hands, that she may the better stay herself during her pains. She being thus placed near the side of her bed, having her midwife at hand, the better to assist as nature may require, let her take courage, and help her pains the best she can, bearing them down when they take her, which she must do by holding in her breath, and forcing them as much as possible, in like manner as when she goes to stool; for by such straining, the diaphragma, or midriff, being strongly thrust downwards, necessarily forces down the womb and the child in it. In the meantime, let the midwife endeavour to comfort her all she can, exhorting her to bear her labour courageously, telling her it will be quickly over, and that there is no fear but she will have a speedy delivery. Let the midwife also, having no rings on her fingers, anoint them with oil or fresh butter, and therewith dilate gently the inward orifice of the womb, putting her finger ends into the entry thereof, and then stretch them one from the other, when her pains take her; by this means endeavouring to help forward the child, and thrusting, by little and little, the sides of the orifice towards the hinder part of the child's head, anointing it with fresh butter, if it be necessary.

When the head of the infant is a little advanced into the inward orifice, the midwives' phrase is, "It is crowned;" because it girds and surrounds it just as a crown; but when it is so far that the extremities begin to appear without the privy parts, they then say, "The child is in the passage;" and at this time the women feels herself as it were scratched, or pricked with pins, and is ready to imagine that the midwife hurts her, when it is occasioned by the violent distention of these parts, and the laceration which sometimes the bigness of the child's head causeth there. When things are in this posture, let the midwife seat herself conveniently to receive the child, which will now come quickly, and with her finger ends (which she must be sure to keep close paired) let her endeavour to thrust the crowning of the womb (of which I have spoken before) back over the head of the child; and as soon as it is advanced as far as the ears or thereabouts, let her take hold of the two sides with her two hands, that when a good pain comes she may quickly draw forth the child, taking care that the navel-string be not entangled about the neck, or any other part, as sometimes it is, lest thereby the after-burden be pulled with violence, and perhaps the womb also, to which it is fastened, and so either cause her to flood, or else break the strings, both which are of bad consequence to the woman, whose delivery may thereby be rendered the more difficult. It must also be carefully observed, that the head be not drawn forth straight, but shaking it a little from one side to the other, that the shoulders may sooner and easier take their place immediately after it is past, without losing any time, lest, the head being past, the child be stopt there by the largeness of the shoulders, and so come in danger of being suffocated and strangled in the passage, as it sometimes happens, for the want of care therein. But as soon as the head is born, if there be need, she may slide her fingers under the armpits, and the rest of the body will follow without any difficulty.

As soon as the midwife hath in this manner drawn forth the child, let her put it on one side, lest the blood and water, which follow immediately, should do it an injury, by running into its mouth and nose as they would do if it lay on its back, and so endanger the choaking of it. The child being thus born, the next thing requisite is to bring away the after-burden: but before that, let the midwife be very careful to examine whether there be more children in the womb: for sometimes a woman may have twins that expected it not; which the midwife may easily know, by the continuance of the pains after the child is born, and the bigness of the mother's belly. But the midwife may be more sure of it, if she puts her hand up to the entry of the womb, and finds there another water gathering, and a child in it presenting to the passage: and if she finds it so, she must have a care of going to fetch the after-birth, till the woman be delivered of all the children she is pregnant with. Wherefore the first string must be cut, being first tied with a thread three or four double, and fasten the other end with a string to the woman's thighs, to prevent the inconvenience it may cause by hanging between her thighs; and then, removing the child already born, she must take care to deliver her of the rest, observing all the same circumstances as with the first; after which it will be necessary to fetch away the after-birth or births. But of that I shall treat in another section; and first show what is to be done to the new-born infant.

SECTION II.

Of the Cutting of the Child's Navel String.

Though this is by many accounted but a trifle, yet great care is to be taken about it; and it shows none of the least art and skill of a midwife to do it as it should be; and that it may be so done, the midwife ought to observe, 1. The time. 2. The place. 3. The manner. 4. The event.

1. The time is, as soon as ever the infant comes out of the womb, whether it brings part of the after-birth with it or not; for sometimes the child brings into the world a piece of the amnios upon its head, and is what midwives call the *caul*, and ignorantly attribute some extraordinary virtue to the child that is so born; but this opinion is only the effect of their ignorance; for when the child is born with such a crown (as some call it) upon its brows, it generally betokens weakness, and denotes a short life. But to proceed to the matter in hand. As soon as the child is come into the world, it should be considered whether it is weak or strong: and if it be

weak, let the midwife gently put back part of the vital and natural blood into the body of the child by its navel; for that recruits a weak child (the vital and natural spirits being communicated by the mother to the child by its navel-string; but if the child be strong, the operation is needless. Only let me advise you, that many children that are born seemingly dead, may be soon brought to life again, if you squeeze six or seven drops of blood out of that part of the navel-string which is cut off, and give it to the child inwardly.

2. As to the place in which it should be cut, that is, whether it should be cut long or short, it is that which authors can scarcely agree in, and which many midwives quarrel about; some prescribing it to be cut at four fingers breadth, which is at best, but an uncertain rule, unless all fingers were of one size. It is a received opinion, that the parts adapted to generation are contracted or dilated according to the cutting of the navel-string; and this is the reason why midwives are generally so kind to their own sex, that they leave a longer part of the navel-string of a male than a female, because they would have the males provided for the encounter of Venus; and the reason they give, why they cut that of females shorter is, because they believe it makes them modest, and their privities narrower, which makes them more acceptable to their husbands. Mizaldus was not altogether of the opinion of these midwives, and he therefore ordered the navel-string to be cut long both in male and female children; for which he gives this reason, that the instrument of generation follows the proportion of it; and therefore, if it be cut too short in a female, it will be a hinderance to her having children. I will not go about to contradict the opinions of Mizaldus: these experience has made good:—The one is, that if the navel-string of a child, after it is cut, be suffered to touch the ground, the child will never hold its water either sleeping or waking but will be subject to an involuntary making of water all its lifetime. The other is, that a piece of the child's navel-string carried about one, so that it touch his skin, defends him that wears it from the falling sickness and convulsions.

3. As to the manner it must be cut: let the midwife take a brown thread, four or five times double, of an ell long, or thereabouts, tied with a single knot at each of the ends, to prevent their entangling; and with this thread so accommodated (which the midwife must have in readiness before the woman's labour, as also a good pair of scissors, that so no time may be lost) let her tie the string within an inch of the belly with a double knot, and, turning about the end of the thread, let her tie two more on the other side of the string, reiterating it again, if it be necessary; then let her cut off

the navel another inch below the ligatures, towards the afterbirth, so that there only remains but two inches of the string, in the midst of which will be the knot we speak of, which must be so strait knit as not to suffer a drop of blood to squeeze out of the vessels; but care must be taken, not to knit it so strait as to cut it in two, and therefore, the thread must be pretty thick, and pretty strait cut, it being better too strait than too lose; for some children have miserably lost their lives, with all their blood, before it was discovered, because the navel-string was not well tied; therefore great care must be taken that no blood squeeze through; for if there do, a new knot must be made with the rest of the string. You need not fear to bind the navel-string very hard, because it is void of sense, and that part of it which you leave falls off of its own accord in a very few days, sometimes in six or seven, or sooner, but never tarries longer than eight or nine. When you have thus cut the navel-string, then take care the piece that falls off touch not the ground, for the reason I told you Mizaldus gave, which experience has justified.

4. The last thing I mentioned was, the event or consequence, or what follows cutting the navel-string. As soon as the navel-string is cut off, apply a little cotton or lint to the place to keep it warm, lest the cold enter into the body of the child, which it most certainly will do, if you have not bound it hard enough. If the lint or cotton you apply to it be dipped in oil of roses, it will be the better; and then put another rag three or four times double upon the belly; upon the top of all, put another small bolster; and then swathe it with a linen swathe, four fingers broad, to keep it steady, lest by moving too much, or by being continually stirred from side to side, it comes to fall off before the navel-string which you left remaining is fallen off. It is the usual custom of midwives to put a piece of burnt rag to it, which we commonly call tinder; but I would rather advise them to put a litte ammoniac to it, because of its drying quality.

SECTION III.

How to bring away the After-burden.

A Woman cannot be said to be fairly delivered, though the child be born, till the after-burden be also taken from her; herein differing from most animals, who, when they have brought forth their young, cast forth nothing else but some water, and the membranes which contained them. But women have an after-labour, which sometimes proves more dangerous than the first; and how to bring it safely away, without prejudice to her, shall be my business to show in this section.

As soon as the child is born, before the midwife either ties or cuts the navel-string, lest the womb should close, let her take the string and wind it once or twice about one or two of the fingers of her left hand joined together, the better to hold it, with which she may draw it moderately, and with the right hand she may only take a single hold of it above the left near the privities, drawing likewise with that very gently, resting the while the fore-finger of the same hand, extended and stretched forth along the string towards the entry of the vagina, always observing, for the greater facility, to draw it from the side where the burden cleaves least; for, in so doing, the rest will separate the better: and special care must be taken that it be not drawn forth with too much violence, lest by breaking the string near the burden the midwife be obliged to put the whole hand into the womb to deliver the woman; and she needs to be a very skilful person that undertakes it, lest the womb, to which this burden is sometimes very strongly fastened, be drawn away with it, as it has sometimes happened. It is therefore best to use such remedies as may assist nature. And here take notice, that what brings away the birth, will also bring away the after-birth. And therefore, for effecting this work, I will lay down the following rules.

1. Use the same means in bringing away the after-birth that you made use of to bring away the birth; for the same care and circumspection are needful now that were then.

2. Considering the labouring woman cannot but be much spent by what she has already undergone in bringing forth the infant; and therefore be sure to give her something to comfort her. And in this case good jelly-broths, also a little wine and toast in it, and other comforting things, will be very necessary.

3. A little white hellebore in powder, to make her sneeze, is in this case very proper.

4. Tansey and the stone Ætites, applied as before directed, are also of good use in this case.

5. If you take the herb vervain, and either boil it in wine, or make a syrup with the juice of it, which you may do by adding to it double its weight of sugar, (having clarified the juice before you boil it,) a spoonful of that given to the woman is very efficacious to bring away the secundine; and featherfew and mugwort have the same operation, taken as the former.

6. Alexander boiled in wine, and the wine drank, also

sweet cervile, sweet cicely, angelica roots, and musterwort, are excellent remedies in this case.

7. Or, if this fail, the smoke of marigolds, received up a woman's privities by a funnel, have been known to bring away the after-birth, even when the midwife let go her hold.

8. Boil mugwort in water till it be very soft; then take it out and apply it in the manner of a poultice to the navel of the labouring woman, and it instantly brings away the birth and after-birth. But special care must be taken to remove it as soon as they come away, lest by its longer tarrying it should draw away the womb also.

SECTION IV.

Of Laborious and Difficult Labours, and how the Midwife is to proceed therein.

THERE are three sorts of bad labours, all painful and difficult, but not all properly unnatural. It will be necessary therefore to distinguish these.

The *first* of these labours is that wherein the mother and child suffer very much by extreme pain and difficulty, even though the child come right: and this is distinguishably called the laborious labour.

The *second* is that which is difficult, and differs not much from the former, except that, besides those extraordinary pains, it is generally attended with some unhappy accident, which, by retarding the birth, causes the difficulty; but these difficulties being removed, it accellerates the birth and hastens the delivery.

Some have asked, what is the reason that women bring forth their children with so much pain? I answer, the sense of feeling is distributed to the whole body by the nerves; and the mouth of the womb being so strait that it must of necessity be dilated at the time of the woman's delivery, the dilating thereof stretches the nerves, and from thence comes pain. And therefore the reason why some women have more pain in their labours than others proceeds from their having the mouth of the matrix more full of nerves than others.

The best way to remove those difficulties that occasion hard pains and labour is to show first from whence they proceed. Now the difficulty of labour proceeds either from the mother, or child, or both.

From the mother, by reason of the indisposition of the body, or from some particular part only, and chiefly the womb, as when the womb is weak, and the mother is not active to expel its burden, or from weakness or disease, or want of spirits; or it may be from some strong passion of the mind with which she was before possessed; she may also be too young, and so may have the passage too strait; or too old, and then, if it be her first child, because her pains are too dry and hard, and cannot be easily dilated, as happens also to them which are too lean; likewise those who are either small, short, or deformed, as crooked women, who have not a breast strong enough to help their pains, and to bear them down, and persons that are crooked having sometimes the bones of the passage not well shaped. The cholic also hinders labour, by preventing the true pains; and all great and acute pains, as when the woman is taken with a violent fever, a great flooding, frequent convulsions, bloody flux, or any other great distemper. Also, excrements retained, cause much difficulty, and so does a stone in the bladder; or when the bladder is full of urine, without being able to void it; or when the woman is troubled with great and painful biles. It may also be from the passages, when the membranes are thick, the orifice too strait, and the neck of the womb not sufficiently open, the passages pressed and strained by tumours in the adjacent parts, or when the bones are too firm, and will not open, which very much endangers the mother and child; or when the passages are not slippery, by reason of the waters having broke too soon, or of the membranes being too thin. The womb may be also out of order with respect to its bad situation, or conformation, having its neck too strait, hard, and callous, which may easily be so naturally, or may come by accident, being many times caused by a tumour, an imposthume, ulcer, or superfluous flesh.

As to hard labour occasioned by the child, it is when the child happens to stick to a mole, or when it is so weak it cannot break the membranes; or if it be too big all over, or in the head only, or if the navel vessels are twisted about its neck; when the belly is hydropical; or when it is monstrous, having two heads, or joined to another child; also, when the child is dead, or so weak that it can contribute nothing to its birth; likewise when it comes wrong: or when there are two or more. And to all these various difficulties there is oftentimes one more, and that is, the ignorance of the midwife, who, for want of understanding in her business, hinders nature in her work instead of helping her.

Having thus looked into the causes of hard labour, I will now show the industrious midwife how she may minister some relief to the labouring woman under these difficult circumstances. But it will require understanding and judgment to the midwife, when she finds a woman in difficult labour, to know the particular obstruction, or cause thereof, that so a suitable remedy may be applied; as, for instance, when it happens by the mother's being too young and too strait, she must be gently treated, and the passages anointed with oil, hog's lard, or fresh butter, to relax and dilate them the easier, lest there should happen a rupture of any part when the child is born, for sometimes the peritoneum breaks, with the skin from the privities of the fundament.

But if the woman be in years with her first child, let her lower parts be anointed to mollify the inward orifice, which, in such a case being more hard and callous, does not easily yield to the distention of labour, which is the true cause why such women are longer in labour, and also why their children, being forced against the inward orifice of the womb (which, as I have said, is a little callous) are born with great humps and bruises on their heads.

Those women that are very small and misshapen, should not be put to bed, at least, till their waters are broke, but rather kept upright, and assisted to walk about the chamber, by being supported under the arms; for, by that means, they will breathe more freely, and mend their pains better than on the bed, because there they lie all on a heap. As for those that are very lean, and have hard labour from that cause, let them moisten the parts with oils and ointments, to make them more smooth and slippery, that the head of the infant and the womb be not so compressed and bruised by the hardness of the mother's bones which form the passage. If the cause be weakness, she ought to be strengthened, the better to support her pains; to which end give her good jelly broths, and a little wine with a toast in it. If she fears her pains, let her be comforted, assuring her that she will not endure many more, but be delivered in a little time. But if her pains be slow and small, or none at all, they must be provoked by frequent and pretty strong clysters; let her walk about the chamber, that so the weight of the child may help them forward. If she flood or have strong convulsions, she must then be helped by a speedy delivery; the operation I shall relate in the section of unnatural labours. If she be costive, let her use clysters, which may also help to dispel the cholic, at those times very injurious, because attended with useless pains, and because such bear not downward, and so help not to forward the birth. If she find no obstruction or stoppage of the urine, by reason the womb bears too much on the bladder, let her lift up her belly a little with her hand, and try if by that she receives any benefit; if she find she does not, it will be necessary to introduce a catheter into her bladder, and thereby draw forth her urine. If the difficulty be from the ill posture of the woman, let her be placed otherwise, in a posture more suitable and convenient for her; also if it proceed from the indispositions of the womb, as from its oblique situation, &c., it must be remedied, as well as it can be, by the placing her body accordingly; or, if it be a vicious conformation, having the neck too hard, too callous, and too strait, it must be anointed with oils and ointment, as before directed. If the membranes be so strong as that the waters do not break in due time, they may be broken with the fingers, if the midwife be first well assured that the child is come forward into the passage, and ready to follow presently after; or else, by the breaking of the waters too soon, the child may be in danger of remaining dry a long time: to supply which defect, you may moisten the parts with fomentations, decoctions, and emollient oils: which is not half so well as when nature does her work in her own time, with the ordinary slime and waters. These membranes do sometimes press forth with the waters three or four fingers' breadth out of the body before the child, resembling a bladder full of water: but there is then no great danger to break them, if they be not already broken; for when the case is so, the child is always in readiness to follow, being in the passage; but let the midwife be very careful not to pull it with her hand, lest the after-burden be thereby loosened before its time, for it adheres thereto very strongly. If the navel-string happen to come first, it must presently be put up again, and kept so if possible, or otherwise the woman must immediately be delivered. But if the after-burden should come first, it must not be put up again by any means: for the infant having no further occasion for it, it would be but an obstacle if it were put up: in this case it must be cut off, having tied the navel-string, and afterwards drawn forth the child with all the speed that may be, lest it be suffocated.

SECTION V.

Of Women labouring with a dead Child.

WHEN the difficulty of labour arises from a dead child, it is a case of great danger to the mother, and great care ought to be taken therein; but before any thing be done, the midwife ought to be well assured the child is dead indeed, which may be known by these signs.

1. The breast suddenly slacks, or falls flat, or bags down. 2. A great coldness possesses the belly of the mother, especially about the navel. 3. Her urine is thick, and a filthy stinking settles at the bottom. 4. No motion of the child can be perceived; for the trial whereof, let the midwife put her hand in warm water, and lay it upon her belly; for that, if it is alive, will make it stir. 5. She is very subject to dream of dead men, and be affrighted therewith. 6. She has extravagant longings to eat such things as are contrary to nature. 7. Her breath stinks, though not used so to do. 8. When she turns herself in her bed, or rises up, the child sways that way like a lump of lead.

These things being carefully observed, the midwife may make a judgment whether the child be alive or dead, especially if the woman take the following prescription: "Take half a pint of white wine and burn it, and add thereto half an ounce of cinnamon, but no other spices whatever; and when she has drank it, if her travailing pains come upon her, the child is certainly dead; but if not, the child may possibly be either weak or sick, but not dead; this will bring her pains upon her if it be dead, and will refresh the child, and give her ease, if it be living; for cinnamon refresheth and strengtheneth the child.

Now if, upon trial, it be found the child is dead, let the mother do all she can to forward the delivery, because a dead child can be nowise helpful therein. It will be necessary, therefore, that she take some comfortable things to prevent her fainting, by reason of the putrid vapours ascending from the dead child. And in order to her delivery, let her take the following herbs boiled in white wine (or at least as many of them as you can get,) viz. dittany, betony, pennyroyal, sage, featherfew, centaury, ivy leaves, and berries. Let her also take sweet bazil, in powder, and half a dram at a time, in white wine; let her privities be also anointed with the juice of the garden-tansey. Or take the tansey in the summer, when it can be most plentifully had, and before it runs up to the flower, and having bruised it well, boil it in oil till the juice of it be consumed. If you set it in the sun, after you have mixed it with oil, it will be more effectual. This an industrious midwife, who would be prepared against all events, ought to have always by her. As to the manner of her delivery, the same methods must be used as are mentioned in the section of natural labour. And here I cannot but commend again the stone Ætites, held near the privities, whose magnetic virtue renders it exceedingly necessary on this occasion, for it draws the child any way, with the same facility that the loadstone draws iron.

Let the midwife also make a strong decoction of hyssop with water, and let the woman drink it very hot, and it will in a little time bring away the dead child.

If, as soon as she is delivered of the dead child, you are in doubt that part of the after-birth is left behind in the body (for in such cases as these, many times, it rots, and comes away piece-meal,) let her continue drinking the same decoction till her body be cleansed.

A decoction made of the herb muster-wort, used as you did the decoction of hyssop, works the same effect. Let the midwife also take roots of pollodum, and stamp them well; warm them a little, and bind them on the sides of her feet, and it will soon bring away the child either dead or alive.

The following medicines likewise are such as stir up the expulsive faculty; but in this case they must be made stronger, because the motion of the child ceaseth.

Take savine, round birthwort, trochisks of myrrh, afaram roots, cinnamon, saffron, each half a dram; make a powder, give a dram.

Or she may purge first, and then apply an emollient, anointing her about the womb with oil of lilies, sweet almonds, camomile, hen and goose grease. Also foment to get out the child with a decoction of mercury, orris, wild cucumbers, sæcus, broom flowers. Then anoint the privities and loins with ointment of sowbread. Or,

Take coloquintida, agaric, birthwort, of each a dram; make a powder; add ammoniacum dissolved in wine, ox gall each two drams; with oil of keir make an ointment. Or this pessary:—

Take birthwort, orris, black hellebore, coloquintida, myrrh, each a dram; powdered amoniacum dissolved in wine, ox gall, each two drams. Or make a fume with an ass's hoof burnt, or gallianum, or castor, and let it be taken in with a funnel.

To take away pains, and strengthen the parts, foment with the decoction of mugwort, mallows, rosemary, with wood myrtle, St. John's wort, each half an ounce, spermaceti two drams, deers suet an ounce; with wax make an ointment. Or,

Take wax six ounces, spermaceti an ounce; melt them, dip flax therein, and lay it all over her belly.

If none of these things will do, the last remedy is to use surgery, and then the midwife ought without delay to send for an expert and able man-midwife, to deliver her by manual operation; of which I shall treat more in the next chapter.

CHAPTER VI.

Of Unnatural Labours.

In showing the duty of a midwife, when the childbearing woman's labour is unnatural, it will be requisite to show, in the first place, what I mean by unnatural labour; for, for women to bring forth children in pain and sorrow is natural to all. Therefore, that which I call unnatural is, when the child comes to the birth in a contrary posture to that which nature ordained, and in which the generality of children come into the world.

The right and natural birth is, when the child comes with its head first, and yet this is too short a definition of a natural birth; for if any part of the head but the crown comes first, so that the body follows not in a straight line, it is a wrong and difficult birth, even though the head comes first. Therefore, if the child come with its feet first, or with the side across, it is quite contrary to nature, or to speak more plainly, that which I call unnatural.

Now, there are four general ways a child may come wrong, 1. When any of the fore parts of the body first present themselves. 2. When, by any unhappy transportation, any of the hinder parts of the body first present themselves. 3. When either of the sides, or, 4, the feet present themselves first. To these the different wrong postures that a child can present itself may be reduced.

SECTION I.

How to deliver a Woman of a dead Child by Manual Operation.

When manual operation is necessary, let the operator acquaint the woman of the absolute necessity there is for such an operation, and that, as the child has already lost its life, there is no other way left for the saving of hers. Let him also inform her, for her encouragement, that he doubts not, with the divine blessing, to deliver her safely; and that the pain arising thereby will not be so great as she fears. Then let him endeavour to stir up the woman's pains by giving her some sharp clyster, to excite her throws to bear down and bring forth the child. And if this prevail not, let him proceed with the manual operation.

First, therefore, let her be placed across the bed that he may operate the easier, and let her lie on her back, with her hips a little higher than her head, or at least the body equally placed, when it is necessary to put back or turn the infant to give it a better posture. Being thus situated, she must fold her legs so as her heels be towards her buttocks, and her thighs spread, and held so by a couple of strong persons: there must be others also to support her under her arms, that the body may not slide down when the child is drawn forth; for which, sometimes, a great strength is required. Let the sheets and blankets cover her thighs, for decency's sake, and with respect to the assistance, and also to prevent her catching cold; the operator here governing himself as well with respect to his convenience, and the facility and surety of the operation, as to other things. Then let him anoint the entrance of the womb with oil or fresh butter, if necessary, that so with more ease he may introduce his hand, which must also be anointed; and having, by the signs before mentioned, received satisfaction that it is a dead child, he must do his endeavour to fetch it away as soon as he possibly can. If the child offer the head first, he must gently put it back, until he hath liberty to introduce his hand quite into the womb; then sliding it along, under the belly, to find the feet, let him draw it forth by them, being very careful to keep the head from being locked in the passage, and that it be not separated from the body: which may be effected the more easily, because the child being very rotten and putrified, the operator needs not be so mindful to keep the breast and face downwards as he is in living births. But if, notwithstanding all these precautions, by reason of the child's putrefaction, the head should be separated and left behind in the womb, it must be drawn forth according to the directions which shall be given in section third of this chapter. But when the head, coming first, is so far advanced that it cannot well be put back, it is better to draw it forth so, than to torment the woman too much by putting it back to turn it and bring it by the feet: but the head being a part round and slippery, it may so happen that the operator cannot take hold of it with his fingers by reason of its moisture, nor put them up to the side of it, because the passage is filled with its bigness; he must therefore take a proper instrument, and put it up as far as he can, without violence, between the womb and the child's head, observing to keep the point of it towards the head (for the child being dead before, there can be no danger in the operation,) and let him fasten it there, giving it good hold upon one of the bones of the skull, that it may not slide, and after it is well fixed in the head, he may therewith draw it forth, keeping the ends of the fingers of his left hand flat upon the opposite side, the better to help to disengage it, and by wagging it a little, to conduct it directly out of the passage, until the head be quite born; and then taking hold of it with the hands only, the shoulders may be drawn into the passage, and so sliding the fingers of both hands under the arm-pits, the child may be quite delivered; and then the after-burden fetched, to finish the operation, being careful not to pluck the navel-string too hard, lest it break, as often happens, when it is corrupt.

If the dead child come with the arm up the shoulder so extremely swelled that the woman must suffer too great violence to have it put back, it is then (being first well assured the child is dead) best to take it off by the shoulder joints, by twisting it three or four times about, which is very easily done by reason of the softness and tenderness of the body. After the arm is so separated, and no longer possesses the passage, the operator will have more room to put up his hand into the womb, to fetch the child by the feet, and bring it away.

But although the operator be sure the child is dead in the womb, yet he must not therefore presently use instruments, because they are never used but when hands are not sufficient, and there is no other remedy to prevent the woman's danger, or to bring forth the child any other way; and the judicious operator will choose that way which is the least hazardous and most safe.

SECTION II.

How a Woman must be delivered, when the Child's Feet come first.

THERE is nothing more obvious to those whose business it is to assist labouring women, than that the several unnatural postures in which children present themselves at their birth are the occasions of most of the bad labours and ill accidents that happen unto them in that condition.

And since midwives are very often obliged, because of the unnatural situations, to draw the children forth by the feet, I conceive it to be proper first to show how a child must be brought forth that presents itself in that posture, because it will be a guide to several of the rest.

I know indeed that in this case it is the advice of several authors to change the figure, and place the head so that it may present to the birth; and this counsel I should be very inclinable to follow, could they but also show how it may be done. But it will appear very difficult, if not impossible, to be performed, if we would avoid the danger that by such violent agitations both the mother and the child must be put into; and therefore my opinion is, that it is better to draw forth by the feet, when it presents itself in that posture, than to venture a worse accident by turning it.

As soon, therefore, as the waters are broken, and it is known that the child comes thus, and that the womb is open enough to admit the midwife's or operator's hand into it, (or else by anointing the passage with oil or hog's grease, to endeavour to dilate it by degrees, using her fingers to this purpose, spreading them one from the other, after they are together entered, and continuing to do so till they be sufficiently dilated,) then, taking care that her nails be well pared, no rings on her fingers, and the woman placed in the manner directed in the former section, let her gently introduce her hand into the entrance of the womb, where, finding the child's feet, let her draw it forth in the manner I shall presently direct; only let her first see whether it presents one foot or both; and if but one foot, she ought to consider whether it be the right foot or left, and also in what fashion it comes; for, by that means, she will soon come to know where to find the other, which, as soon as she knows and finds, let her very gently draw it forth with the other; but of this circumstance she must be especially careful, viz. that the second be not the foot of another child—for, if so, it may be of the most fatal consequence, for she may sooner split both mother and child, than draw them forth: but this may be easily prevented, if she but slide the hand up by the first leg and thigh to the twist, and there find both thighs joined together, and descending from one and the same body. And this is also the best means to find the other foot when it comes but with one.

As soon as the midwife has found both the child's feet, she may draw them forth, and holding them together, may bring them by little and little in this manner; taking afterwards hold of the arms and thighs as soon as she can come at them, drawing them so till the hips come forth. While this is doing, let her observe to wrap the parts in a single cloth, that so her hands, being always g easy, slide not on the infant's body, which is very slippery, because of the vicious humours which are all over it, and prevent one's taking good hold of it; which being done, she may take hold under the hips, so as to draw it forth to the beginning of the breast; and let her on both sides with her hand bring down the child's hand along its body, which she may easily find; and then let her take care that the belly and face of the child be downwards: for, if they should be upwards, there would be some danger of its being stopped by the chin over the share bone: and therefore, if it be not so, she must turn it to that posture: which may be easily done, if she takes a proper hold of the body when the breast and arms are forth, in the manner we have said, and draws it, turning it in proportion on that side which it most inclines to, till it be turned with the face downwards: and so, having brought it to the shoulders, let her lose no time, desiring the woman at the same time to bear down, that so drawing, the head at that instant may take its place, and not be stopped in the passage. Some children there are whose heads are so big, that when the whole body is born, yet that stops the passage, though the midwife takes all possible care to prevent it. And when this happens, she must endeavour to draw forth the child by the shoulders, taking care that she separate not the body from the head, as I have known it done by the midwife, discharging it by degrees from the bones in the passage with the fingers of each hand, sliding them on each side opposite the one to the other, sometimes above, and sometimes under, until the work be ended: endeavouring to despatch it as soon as possible, lest the child be suffocated, as it will unavoidably be if it remain long in that posture: and this being well and carefully effected, she may soon after fetch away the after-birth, as I have before directed.

SECTION III.

How to bring away the Head of the Child, when separated from the Body, and left behind in the Womb.

Though the utmost care be taken in bringing away the child by the feet, yet, if it happen to be dead, it is sometimes so putrified and corrupt, that with the least pull the head separates from the body, and remains alone in the womb, and cannot be brought away but with a manual operation and great difficulty, it being extremely slippery, by reason of the place where it is, and from the roundness of its figure, on which no hold can be well taken; and so very great is the difficulty in this case, that sometimes two or three able practitioners in midwifery have, one after the other, left the operation unfinished, as not able to effect it, after the utmost efforts of their industry, skill, and strength; so that the woman, not being able to be delivered, perished. To prevent which fatal accident let the following operation be observed.

When the infant's head separates from the body, and is left alone behind, whether through putrefaction or otherwise, let the operator immediately, without any delay, while the womb is yet open, direct up his right hand to the mouth of the head (for no other hole can there be had,) and having found it, let him put one or two of his fingers into it, and the thumb under its chin, then let him draw it by little and little, holding it by the jaws: but if that fails, as sometimes it will, when putrified then let him pull forth the right hand, and slide up his left with which he must support the head, and with the right let him take a narrow instrument, called a *crochet*, but let it be strong and with a single branch, which he must guide along the inside of his hand, with the point of it towards it, for fear of hurting the womb: and having thus introduced it, let him turn it towards the head, to strike either in an eyehole, or the hole of an ear, or behind the head, or else between the suture, as he finds it most convenient and easy, and then draw forth the head so fastened with the said instrument, still helping to conduct it with the left hand; but when he hath brought it near the passage, being strongly fastened to the instrument, let him remember to draw forth his hand, that the passage not being filled with it, may be larger and easier, keeping still a finger or two on the side of the head, the better to disengage it.

There is also another method, with more ease and less hardship than the former: let the operator take a soft fillet or linen slip, of about four fingers' breadth, and the length of three quarters of an ell, or thereabouts; taking the two ends with the left hand, and the middle with the right, and let him so put it up with his right as that it may be beyond the head, to embrace it as a sling doth a stone, and afterwards draw forth the fillet by the two ends together; it will thus be easily drawn forth, the fillet not hindering the least passage, because it takes up little or no space.

When the head is fetched out of the womb, care must be taken that not the least part of it be left behind, and likewise to cleanse the woman well of her after-burden, if it remain. If the burden be wholly separated from the sides of the womb, that ought to be first brought away, because it may also hinder the taking hold of the head. But if it still adhere to the womb, it must not be meddled with till the head be brought away; for if one should endeavour to separate it from the womb, it might then cause a flooding, which would be augmented by the violence of the operation; the vessels to which it is joined remaining for the most part open as long as the womb is distended, which the head causeth while it is retained in it, and cannot close till this strange body be voided, and this it doth by contracting and compressing itself together, as has been more fully before explained. Besides, the after-birth remaining thus cleaving to the womb during the operation prevents it from receiving easily either bruise or hurt.

SECTION IV.

How to deliver a Woman when the Child's Head is presented to the Birth.

Though some may think it a natural labour, when the child's head comes first; yet, if the child's head present not the right way, even that is an unnatural labour; and therefore, though the head comes first, yet, if it be the side of the head instead of the crown, it is very dangerous both to the mother and child, for the child's neck would be broken if born in that manner; and by how much the mother's pains continue to bear the child, which is impossible, unless the head be rightly placed, the more the passages are stopped. Therefore, as soon as the position of the child is known, the woman must be laid with all speed, lest the child should advance further into the vicious posture, and thereby render it more difficult to thrust it back, which must be done in order to place the head right in the passage, as it ought to be.

To this purpose, therefore, place the woman so, that her buttocks may be a little higher than her head and shoulders, causing her to lean a little upon the opposite side to the child's ill posture; then let the operator slide up his hand, well anointed with oil, by the side of the child's head to bring it right gently with his fingers between the head, and the womb; but if the head be so engaged that it cannot be done that way, he must then put up his hand to the shoulders that so by thrusting them back a little into the womb, sometimes on the one side and sometimes on the other, he may by little and little give it a natural position. I confess it would be better, if the operator could put back the child by its shoulders with both hands: but the head takes up so much room, that he will find much ado to put up one, with which he must perform this operation, and with the help of the finger ends of the other hand put forth the child's birth, as when the labour is natural.

Some children present their face first, having their heads turned back, in which posture it is extremely difficult for a child to be born; and if it continue so long, the face will be swelled, and become black and blue, so that it will at first seem monstrous, which is occasioned, as well by the compression of it in that place, as by the midwife's fingers handling it, in order to place it in a better posture. But this blackness will wear away in three or four days time by anointing it often with oil of sweet almonds. To deliver the birth, the same operation must be used as in the former, when the child comes first with the side of the head; only let the midwife or operator work very gently, to avoid as much as possible bruising the face.

SECTION V.

How to deliver a Woman when the Child presents one or both Hands together with the head.

SOMETIMES the infant will present some other part together with its head; which if it does, it is usually one or both its hands; and this hinders the birth, because the hands take up part of that passage which is little enough for the head alone: besides that, when this happens, they generally cause the head to lean on one side; and therefore this position may be very well styled unnatural. When the child presents thus, the first thing to be done, after it is perceived, is to prevent it from coming down more, or engaging further in the passage; and therefore the operator having placed the woman on the bed, with her head a little lower than her buttocks, must guide and put back the infant's hand with his own as much as may be, or both of them, if they both come down, to give way to the child's head; and this being done, if the head be on one side, it must be brought into its natural posture, in the middle of the passage, that it may come in a straight line, and then proceed as directed in the foregoing section.

SECTION VI.

How a Woman is to be delivered, when the Hands and Feet of the Infant come together.

THERE are none but will readily grant, that when the hands and feet of an infant present together, the labour must be unnatural; because it is impossible a child can be born in that manner.

In this case, therefore, when the midwife guides her hand to the orifice of the womb, she will perceive only many fingers close together; and if it be not sufficiently dilated, it will be a good while before the hands and feet will be exactly distinguished; for they are sometimes so shut and pressed together, that they seem to be all of one and the same shape; but where the womb is open enough to introduce the hand into it, she will easily know which are the hands and which are the feet: and having taken particular notice thereof, let her slide up her hand, and presently direct it towards the infant's breast which she will find very near, and then let her very gently thrust back the body towards the bottom of the womb, leaving the feet in the same place where she found them: and then having placed the woman in a convenient posture, that is to say, her buttocks a little raised above her breast and head (which situation ought also to be observed when the child is to be put back into the womb,) let the midwife afterwards take hold of the child by the feet, and draw it forth as is directed in the second section.

This labour, though somewhat troublesome, yet is much better than when the child presents only its hands; for then the child must be quite turned about before it can be drawn forth; but in this they are ready, presenting themselves, and there is little to do but to lift and thrust back the upper part of the body, which is almost done of itself, by drawing it by the feet alone.

I confess there are many authors that have written of labours, who would have all wrong births reduced to a natural figure; which is, to turn it that it may come with the head first. But those that have thus written are such as never understood the practical part; for if they had the least experience herein, they would know that it is very often impossible; at least, if it were to be done, that violence must necessarily be used in doing it that would very probably be the death of mother and child in the operation. I would therefore lay down, as a general rule, that whensoever a child presents itself wrong to the birth, in what posture soever, from the shoulders to the feet, it is the best way, and soonest done, to draw it out by the feet; and that it is better to search for them, if they do not present themselves, than try to put it in the natural posture, and place the head foremost: for the great endeavours necessary to be used in turning the infant in the womb do so much weaken both the mother and child, that there remains not afterwards strength enough to commit the operation to the work of nature; for, usually, the woman hath no more throes or pains fit for labour after she has been so wrought upon; for which reason it would be very difficult, and tedious at best, and the child, by such an operation, made very weak, would be in extreme danger of perishing before it could be born. It is therefore much better in these cases to bring it away immediately by the feet; searching for them, as I have already directed, when they do not present themselves; by which the mother will be prevented a tedious labour, and the child be often brought alive into the world, who otherwise could hardly escape death.

SECTION VII.

How a Woman should be Delivered that has Twins, which present themselves in different Postures.

WE have already spoken something of the birth of twins in the chapter of natural labour; for it is not an unnatural labour barely to have twins, provided they come in a right position at the birth. But when they present themselves in different postures; they come properly under the denomination of unnatural labours; and if when one child presents itself in a wrong figure, it makes the labour dangerous and unnatural, it must needs make it much more so when there are several, and render it not only more painful to the mother and children, but to the operator also; for they often trouble each other, and hinder both their births: besides which the womb is so filled with them, that the operator can hardly introduce his hand without much violence, which he must do, if they are to be turned or thrust back, to give them a better position.

When a woman is pregnant with two children, they rarely present to the birth together, the one being generally more forward than the other; and that is the reason that but one is felt, and that many times the midwife knows not that there are twins till the first is born, and that she is going to fetch away the after-birth. In the fifth chapter, wherein I treated of natural labour, I have showed how a woman should be delivered of twins, presenting themselves both right, and therefore, before I close the chapter of unnatural labour, it only remains that I show what ought to be done when they either both come wrong, or one of them only, as for the most part it happens; the first generally coming right, and the second with the feet forward, or in some worse posture. In such a case, the birth of the first must be hastened as much as possible to make way for the second, which is best brought away by the feet, without endeavouring to place it right, because, it has been, as well as its mother, already tired, and weakened by the birth of the first, and there would be greater danger of its death than likelihood of its coming out of the womb that way.

But if, when the first is born naturally, the second should likewise offer its head to the birth, it would be then best to leave nature to finish what she has so well begun; if nature should be too slow in her work, some of those things mentioned in the fourth chapter, to accelerate the birth, may be properly enough applied: and if after that, the second birth should be yet delayed, let a manual operation be deferred no longer: but the woman being properly placed, as has been before directed, let the operator direct his hand gently into the womb to find the feet, and so draw forth the econd child, which will be the more easily effected, because there is a way made sufficiently by the birth of the first: and if the waters of this second child be not broke, as it often happens, yet intending to bring it by the feet, he need not scruple to break the membranes with his fingers; for though, when the birth of a child is left to the operation of nature, it is necessary that the waters should break of themselves, yet when the child is brought out of the womb by art, there is no danger in breaking of them; nay, on the contrary, it becomes necessary, for without the waters are broken, it would be almost impossible to turn the child.

But herein lies principally the care of the operator, that he be not deceived, when either the hands or feet of both children offer themselves together to the birth; in this case he ought well to consider the operation, as, whether they be not joined together, or any way monstrous, and which part belongs to one child, and which to the other, that so they may be fetched one after the other, and not both together, as might be, if it were duly considered: taking the right foot of the one and the left of the other, and so drawing them together, as if they both belonged to one body, because there is a left and right, by which means it would be impossible ever to deliver them. But a skilful operator will easily prevent this, if, having found two or three feet of several children presenting together in the passage, and taking aside two of the forwardest, a right and a left, and sliding his hand along the legs and thighs up to the twist, if forwards, or the buttocks, if backwards, he find they both belong to one body; of which being thus assured, he may begin to draw forth the neerest, without regarding which is the strongest or weakest, bigger or less, living or dead, having put first a little aside that part of the other child which offers to have the more way, and so despatch the first as soon as may be, observing the same rules as if there were but one, that is, keeping the breast and face downwards, with every circumstance directed in that section where the child comes with its feet first, and not fetch the burden till the second child is born. And therefore, when the operator hath drawn forth one child, he must separate it from the burden, having tied and cut the navel-string, and then fetch the other by the feet in the same manner, and afterwards bring away the after-burden with the two strings, as hath been before showed. If the children present any other part than the feet, the operator may follow the same method as directed in the foregoing section, where the several unnatural positions are fully treated of.

CHAPTER VII.

Directions for Child-bearing Women, in their Lying-in.

SECTION I.

How a Woman newly Delivered ought to be ordered.

As soon as she is laid in her bed, let her be placed in it conveniently for ease and rest, which she stands in great need of, to recover herself of the great fatigue she underwent during her travail; and that she may lie the more easily let hands and body be a little raised, that she may breathe more freely, and cleanse the better, especially of that blood which then comes away, that so it may not clot, which being retained causeth great pain.

Having thus placed her in bed, let her take a draught of burnt white wine, having a dram of spermaceti melted therein. The herb vervain is also singularly good for a woman in this condition, boiling it in what she either eats or drinks, fortifying the womb so exceedingly, that it will do it more good in two days than any other thing does in double that time, having no offensive taste. And this is no more than what she stands in need of, for her lower parts being greatly distended till the birth of the infant, it is good to endeavour the prevention of an inflammation there. Let there be also outwardly applied, all over the bottom of the belly and privities, the following anodyne and cataplasm: take two ounces of oil of sweet almonds, and two or three new laid eggs, yolks and whites, stirring them together in an earthen pipkin over hot embers, till they come to the consistence of a poultice; which being spread upon a cloth must be applied to those parts indifferently warm, having first taken away the closure (which was put to her presently after her delivery,) and likewise such clots of blood as were then left. Let this lie on five or six hours, and then renew it again when you see cause.

Great care ought to be taken at first, that if her body be very weak, she be not kept too hot, for extremity of heat weakens nature and dissolves the strength; and whether she be weak or strong, be sure that no cold air comes near her at first; for cold is an enemy to the spermatic parts, and if it get into the womb, it increases the afterpains, and causes swelling in the womb, and hurts the nerves. As to her diet, let it be hot, and let her eat but a little at a time. Let her avoid the light for the first three days, and longer if she be weak, for her labour weakens her eyes exceedingly, by a harmony between the womb and them. Let her also avoid great noise, sadness, and trouble of mind.

If the womb be foul, which may be easily perceived by the impurity of the blood (which will then easily come away in clots or stinking, or if you suspect any of the after-burden to be left behind, which may sometimes happen,) make her drink of featherfew, mugwort, pennyroyal, and mother of thyme, boiled in white wine and sweetened with sugar.

Panado and new laid eggs are the best meat for her at first; of which she may eat often, but not too much at a time And let her nurse use cinnamon in all her meats and drinks, for it generally strengthens the womb.

Let her stir as little as may be, till after the fifth, sixth or seventh day of her delivery, if she be weak; and let her talk as little as possible, for that tends to weaken her very much.

If she goes not well to stool, give a clyster made only with the decoction of mallows and a little brown sugar.

When she hath lain in a week or more, let her use such things as close the womb, of which knotgrass and comfrey are very good; and to them you may add a little polipodium, for it will do her good, both leaves and root being bruised.

SECTION II.

How to remedy those Accidents which a Lying-in Women is subject to.

I. THE first common and usual accident that troubles women in their lying in, is after pains. They proceed from cold and wind contained in the bowels, with which they are easily filled after labour, because then they have more room to dilate than when the child was in the womb, by which they were compressed: and also because nourishment and matter, contained as well in them as in the stomach, have been so confusedly agitated from side to side during the pains of labour, by the throes which always must compress the belly, that they could not be well digested, whence the wind is afterwards generated, and by consequence the gripes, which, the woman feels running into her belly from side to side according as the wind moves more or less, and sometimes likewise from the womb, because of the compression and commotion which the bowels make. These being generally the case, let us now apply a suitable remedy.

1. Boil an egg soft, and pour out the yolk of it: with which mix a spoonful of cinnamon water, and let her drink it: and if you mix in two grains of ambergrise, it will be better; and yet vervain taken in any thing she drinks, will be as effectual as the other.

2. Give the lying-in woman, immediately after delivery, oil of sweet almonds and syrup of maiden hair mixed together. Some prefer oil of walnuts, provided it be made of nuts that are very good; but it tastes worse than the other at best. This will lenify the inside of the intestines by unctuousness, and by that means bring away that which is contained in them more easily.

3. Take and boil onions very well in water, then stamp them with oil of cinnamon, spread them on a cloth, and apply them to the region of the womb.

4. Let her be careful to keep her belly warm, and not drink too cold; and if the pain prove violent, hot clothes, from time to time, must be laid on her belly, or a pancake fried in walnut oil may be applied to it, without swathing her belly too strait. And for the better evacuating the wind out of the intestines, give her a clyster, which may be repeated as often as necessity requires.

5. Take bay berries, beat them to powder, put the powder upon a chafing dish of coals, and let her receive the smoke of them up her privities.

6. Take tar and bear's grease, of each an equal quantity, boil them together, and whilst it is boiling, add a little pigeon's dung to it. Spread some of this upon a linen cloth, and apply it to the reins of the back of her that is troubled with after pains, and it will give her speedy ease.

Lastly. Let her take half a dram of bayberries beaten into a powder in a draught of muscadel or tent.

II. Another accident to which women in childbed are subject is the hemorrhoids, or piles, occasioned through the great straining in bringing the child into the world. To cure this,

1. Let her be let blood in the saphæna vein.

2. Let her use polypodium in her meat and drink, bruised and boiled.

3. Take an onion, and having made a hole in the middle of it, fill it full of oil, roast it, and having bruised it all together, apply it to the fundament.

4. Take a dozen of snails, without shells if you can get them, or else so many shell snails, and pull them out, and having bruised them with a little oil, apply them warm as before.

5. If she go not well to stool, let her take an ounce of cas-

sio fistula drawn at night going to bed; she needs no change of diet after.

III. Retention of the menses is another accident happening to women in childbed; and which is of so dangerous a consequence, that, if not timely remedied, it proves mortal. When this happens,

1. Let the woman take such medicines as strongly provoke the terms, such are dittany, betony, pennyroyal, featherfew, centaury, juniper berries, peony roots.

2. Let her take two or three spoonfulls of briony water each morning.

3. Gentian roots beaten into a powder, and a drain of it taken every morning in wine, are an extraordinary remedy.

4. The roots of birthwort, either long or round, so used and taken as the former, are very good.

5. Take twelve peony seeds, and beat them into a very fine powder, and let her drink them in a draught of hot cardus posset, and let her sweat after And if this last medicine do not bring them down the first time she takes it, let her take as much more three hours after, and it seldom fails.

IV. Overflowing of the menses is another accident incidental to childbed women. For which,

1. Take shepherd's purse, either boiled in any convenient liquor, or dried and beaten in a powder, and it will be an admirable remedy to stop them, this being especially appropriated to the privities.

2. The flowers and leaves of brambles, or either of them, being dried and beaten into powder, and a dram of them taken every morning in a spoonful of red wine, or in a decoction of leaves of the same (which perhaps is much better,) s an admirable remedy for the immoderate flowing of the terms in women.

V. Excoriations, bruises, and rents of the lower part of he womb are often occasioned by the violent distention and separation of the four caruncles in a woman's labour. For he healing of which,

As soon as the woman is laid, if there be only simple contusions and excoriations, then let the anodyne cataplasm, formerly directed, be applied to the lower parts to ease the pain, made of the yolks and whites of new laid eggs and oil of roses, boiled a little over warm embers, continually stirring till it be mixed, and then spread on a fine cloth; it must be applied very warm to the bearing place for five or six hours, and when it is taken away, lay some fine rags dipped in oil of St. John's wort on each side of the bearing place: or let the part excoriated be anointed with oil of St. John's wort twice or thrice a day; also foment the parts with barley water and honey of roses, to cleanse them from the excrements which pass. When the woman makes water, let them be defended with fine rags, and thereby hinder the urine from causing smart and pain.

VI. The curdling and clotting of the milk is another accident that happens to women in childbed; for, in the beginning of childbed, the woman's milk is not purified, because of the great commotions her body suffered during her labour, which affected all the parts, and it is then moved with many humours. Now this clotting of the milk does, for the most part, proceed from the breasts not being fully drawn, and that either because she has too much milk, and that the infant is too small and weak to suck all, or because she doth not desire to be a nurse: for the milk in those cases remaining in the breast after concoction without being drawn loseth the sweetness and the balsamic quality it had, and by reason of the heat it acquires, and the too long stay it makes there, it sours, curdles, and clots, in like manner as we see runnet put into ordinary milk turns it into curds. The curdling of the milk may be also caused by having taken a great cold, and not keeping the breast well covered.

But from what causes soever this curdling of the milk proceeds, the most certain remedy is, speedily to draw the breasts until it is emitted and dried. But in regard that the infant, by reason of weakness, cannot draw strong enough, the woman being hard marked when her milk is curdled, it will be most proper to get another woman to draw her breasts until the milk comes freely, and then she may give her child suck. And that she may not afterwards be troubled with a surplus of milk, she must eat such diet as gives but little nourishment, and keep her body open.

But if the case be such, that the woman neither can nor will be a nurse, it is necessary to apply other remedies for the curing of this distemper: for then it will be best not to draw her breasts: for that will be the way to bring more milk into them. For which purpose, it will be necessary to empty the body, by bleeding the arm: besides which, let the humours be drawn down by strong clysters and bleeding in the foot; nor will it be amiss to purge gently: and to digest, dissolve, and dissipate the curdled milk, apply a cataplasm of pure honey, or that of the four grains dissolved in a decoction of sage, milk, smallage, and fennel, mixing with it oil of camomile, with which oil let the breasts be well anointed. The following liniment is also good to scatter and dissipate the milk.

A Liniment to scatter and dissipate the Milk.

That the milk flowing back to the breast may without offence be dissipated, you must use this ointment: "Take pure wax two ounces, linseed oil half a pound; when the wax is melted, let the liniment be made, wherein linen cloths must be dipped, and according to their largeness, be laid upon the breast; and when it shall be dispersed, and pains no more, let other linen cloths be dipped in the distilled water of acorns, and put upon them."

Note, That the cloths dipped in the distilled water of acorns must be used only by those who cannot nurse their own children: but if a swelling in the breast of her who gives suck do arise, from abundance of milk, and threatens an inflammation, let her use the former ointment, but abstain from using the distilled water of acorns.

CHAPTER VIII.

Directions for the Nurses, in ordering newly born Children.

When the child's navel-string hath been cut, according to the rules before prescribed, let the midwife presently cleanse it from the excrements and filth it brings into the world with it; of which some are within the body, as the urine in the bladder, and the excrement found in the guts; and others without, which are thick, whitish, and clammy, proceeding from the sliminess of the waters. There are children sometimes so covered all over with this, that one would think they were rubbed all over with soft cheese; and some women are of so easy a belief, that they really think it so, because they had some while they were with child. From these excrements, let the child be cleansed with wine and water a little warmed, washing every part therewith, but chiefly the head, because of the hair, also the folds of the groins arm-pits and the cods or privities: which parts must be gently cleansed with a linen rag, or a soft spunge dipped in luke warm wine. If this clammy or vicious excrement stick so close that it will not be easily washed off from those places, it may be fetched off with oil of sweet almonds, or a little fresh butter melted with wine, and afterwards well dried off: also make tents of fine rags, and wetting them in this liquor, clear the ears and nostrils; but for the eyes, wipe them only with a dray soft rag, not dipping it in the wine, lest it should make them smart.

The child being thus washed and cleased from the native blood and impurities which attend it into the world, it must in the next place be searched, to see whether all things be right about it, and that there is no fault or dislocation; whether its nose be straight, or its tongue tied; or whether there be any bruise or tumour of the head; or whether the mould be not overshot; also whether the scrotum (if it be a male) be not blown up and swell'd; and, in short, whether it has suffered any violence by its birth, in any part of its body; and whether all the parts be well and duly shaped; that suitable remedies may be applied, if any thing be found not right. Nor is it enough to see that all be right without, and that the outside of the body be cleansed, but she must chiefly observe whether it dischargeth the excrements contained within, and whether the passage be open; for some have been born without having been perforated: therefore, let her examine whether the conduits of the urine and stool be clear, for want of which some have died, not being able to void their excrements, because timely care was not taken at first. As to the urine all children, as well males as females, do make water as soon as they are born, if they can, especially if they feel the heat of the fire, and sometimes also void the excrements, but not so soon as the urine. If the infant does not ordure the first day, then put up into its fundament a small suppository, to stir it up to be discharged, that it may not cause painful gripes by remaining so long in its belly. A sugar almond may be proper for this purpose, anointed over with a little boiled honey: or else a small piece of Castile soap rubbed over with fresh butter; also give the child for this purpose a little syrup of roses or violets at the mouth, mixed with some oil of sweet almonds drawn without a fire, anointing the belly also with the same oil, or fresh butter.

The midwife having thus washed and cleansed the child, according to the before mentioned directions, let her begin to swaddle it in swathing cloths, and when she dresses the head, let her put small rags behind the ears to dry up the filth which usually engenders there, and so let her do also in the folds of the arm-pits and groins, and so swathe it: then wrap it up warm in a bed with blankets, which there is scarce any woman so ignorant but knows well enough how to do: only let me give them this caution, that they swathe not the child too strait in its blankets, especially about the breast and stomach, that it may breathe the more freely, and not be forced to vomit up the milk it sucks, because the stomach cannot be sufficiently extended to contain it; therefore let its arms and legs, be wrapped in its bed, stretched and strait, and swathed to keep them so, viz. the arms along its sides, and its legs equally both together, with a little of the bed between them, that they may not be galled by rubbing each other; then let the head be kept steady and strait, with a stay fastened on each side of the blanket; and then wrap the child up in mantles and blankets to keep it warm. Let none think this of swathing the infant is needless to set down, for it is necessary it should be thus swaddled to give its little body a strait figure, which is most decent and proper for a man, and to accustom him to keep upon his feet, who otherwise would go upon all-four, as most other animals do.

CHAPTER IX.

SECTION I.

Of Gripes and Pains in the Bellies of Young Children.

This I mention first, as it is often the first and most common distemper which happens to little infants after their birth, many children being so troubled and pained therewith, that it causes them to cry night and day, and at last die of it. The cause of it for the most part comes from the sudden change of their nourishment, for having always received it from the umbilical vessels whilst in the mother's womb, they come on a sudden to change not only the manner of receiving it, but the nature and quality of what they received as soon as they are born: for instead of purified blood only, which was conveyed to them by means of the umbilical vein only, they are now obliged to be nourished with their mother's milk, which they suck with their mouths, and from which are engendered many excrements, causing gripes and pains, and that not only because it is not so pure as the blood with which it was nourished in the womb, but because the stomach and the intestines cannot yet make a good digestion, being unaccustomed to it. It is also caused sometimes by a rough phlegm, and sometimes by worms; for physicians affirm, that worms have been bred in children even in their mother's belly.

Cure. If it proceed from the too sudden changes of nourishment, the remedy must be to forbear giving the child suck for some days, lest the milk be mixed with phlegm, which is then in the stomach corrupt: and at first it must suck but little, until it is accustomed to digest it. If it be the excrements in the intestines, which by their long stay increase these pains, give them at the mouth a little oil of sweet almonds and syrup of roses: if it be worms, lay a cloth dipped in oil of wormwood, mixed with ox gall, upon the belly, or a small cataplasm mixed with the powder of rue, wormwood, coloquintida, aloes, and the seeds of citron incorporated with ox-gall and the powder of lupines. Or give it oil of sweet almonds, with sugar candy, and a scruple of anniseed; it purgeth new born babes from green choler and stinking phlegm; and, if it be given with sugar pap, it allays the griping pains of the belly. Also anoint the belly with oil of dill, or pellitory stamp, with oil of camomile.

SECTION II.

Of Weakness in new-born Infants

WEAKNESS is an accident that many children bring into the world along with them, and is often occasioned by the labour of the mother: by the violence and length whereof they suffer so much, that they are born with great weakness, and many times it is difficult to know whether they are alive or dead, their body appearing so senseless, and their face so blue and livid, that they seem to be quite choaked: and even after some hours, their showing any signs of life is attended with so much weakness, that it looks like a return from death, and that they are still in a dying condition.

CURE. Lay the infant speedily in a warm blanket, and carry it to the fire, and then let the midwife take a little wine in her mouth and spout it into its mouth, repeating it often if there be occasion. Let her apply linen to the breast, and belly, dipped in wine, and let the face be uncovered, that it may breathe the more freely: also, let the midwife keep his mouth a little open, cleanse the nostrils with small linen tents dipped in white wine, so that it may receive the smell of it, and let her chafe every part of its body well with warm cloths, to bring back the blood and spirits, which, being retired inwards, through weakness, often puts it in danger of being choaked. By the application of these means, the infant will gradually recover strength, and begin to stir its limbs by degrees, and at length to cry; and though it be but weakly at first, yet afterwards, as it breathes more freely, its cry will become more strong.

SECTION III.

Of the Fundament being closed up in a newly born Infant.

ANOTHER defect that new-born infants are liable to is to have their fundament closed up; by which they can neither evacuate the new excrements engendered by the milk they suck, nor that which was amassed in their intestines before birth, which is certainly mortal without a speedy remedy. There have been some female children who have had their fundament quite closed, and yet have voided the excrements of the guts by an orifice, which nature, to supply that defect, had made within the neck of the womb.

CURE. Here we must take notice, that the fundament is closed two ways; either by a single skin, through which one may discover some black and blue marks, proceeding from the excrements retained, which, if one touch with the finger, there is a softness felt within, and thereabout it ought to be pierced; or else it is quite stopped by a thick fleshy substance, in such sort that there appears nothing without by which its true situation may be known. When there is nothing but the single skin which makes the closure, the operation is very easy, and the children may do very well; for then an aperture or opening may be made with a small incision knife cross ways, that it may the better receive a round form, and that the place may not afterwards grow together, taking great care not to prejudice the spincter or muscle of the rectum. The incision being thus made, the excrements will certainly have issue. But if, by reason of their long stay in the belly, they become so dry that the infant cannot void them, then let a clyster be given to moisten and bring them away; afterwards put a linen tent into the new made fundament, which at first had best be anointed with honey of roses, and towards the end with a drying cicatrizing ointment, such as unguentum album, or pomphilix, obsearving to cleanse the infant of his excrements, and dry him again as soon and as often as he evacuates them, that so the aperture may be prevented from turning into a malignant ulcer.

But if the fundament be stopped up in such a manner, that neither mark nor appearance of it can be seen or felt, then the operation is much more difficult; and even when it is done, the danger is much greater that the infant will not survive it. Then, if it be a female, and it sends forth its excrements by the way I have mentioned before, it is better not to meddle, than, by endeavouring to remedy an inconvenience, run an extreme hazard of the infant's death. But when there is no vent for the excrements, without which death is unavoidable, then the operation is justifiable.

OPERATION. Let the operator, with a small incision knife that hath but one edge, enter into the void place, and turning the back of it upwards within half a finger's breadth from the child's rump, which is the place where he will certainly find the intestine, let him thrust it forward, that it may be open enough to give free vent to the matter there contained, being especially careful of the sphincter: after which, let the wound be dressed according to the method directed.

SECTION IV.

Of the Thrush, or Ulcers in the Mouth of an Infant.

THE thrush is a distemper that children are very often subject to, and it arises from bad milk, or from foul humour in the stomach; for sometimes, though there be no ill quality in the milk itself, yet it may corrupt in the child's stomach because of its weakness, or some other indisposition: in which, acquiring an acrimony instead of being well digested, there arise from thence biting vapours, which forming a thick viscosity, do thereby produce this distemper.

CURE. It is often difficult, as physicians tell us, because it is seated in hot and moist places, where the putrefaction is easily augmented, and because the remedies applied cannot lodge there, being soon washed away with spittle. But if it arises from too hot quality in the nurse's milk, care must be taken to temper and cool; prescribing her cool diet, bleeding and purging her also, if there be occasion.

Take lentiles husked, powder them, and lay a little of them upon the child's gums. Or take bdellium flower half an ounce, and with oil of roses make a liniment. Also wash the child's mouth with barley and plantain-water, and honey of roses, or syrup of dry roses, mixing with them a little verjuice of lemons, as well to loosen and cleanse the vicious humours which cleave to the inside of the child's mouth, as to cool those parts which are already over-heated. This may be done by means of a small fine rag fastened to the end of a little stick, and dipped therein, whereby the ulcers may be gently rubbed, being careful not to put the child to too much pain, lest an inflammation make the distemper worse. The child's body must also be kept open, that the humours being carried to the lower parts, the vapours may not ascend, as it is usual for them to do when the body is costive and the excrements too long retained.

If the ulcers appear malignant, let such remedies be used to do their work speedily, that the evil qualities that cause them being thereby instantly corrected, their malignity may be prevented: and in this case touch the ulcers with plantain-water, sharpened with the spirits of vitriol: for the remedy must be made sharp, according to the malignity of the distemper. It will be necessary to purge these ill humours out of the whole habit of the child, by giving half an ounce of succory with rhubarb.

SECTION V.

Of Pains in the Ears, Inflammation, Moisture, &c.

The brain in infants is very moist, and hath many excrements which nature cannot send out at its proper passages; they got often to the ears, and there cause pains, flux of blood, with inflammation, and matter, with pain: this in children is hard to be known, as they have no other way to make it known but by constant crying: you will perceive them ready to feel their ears themselves, but will not let others touch them if they can prevent it: and sometimes you may discern the parts about the ears to be very red.

These pains, if let alone, are of dangerous consequences, because they may bring forth watching and epilepsy: for the moisture breeds worms there, and fouls the spongy bones, and by degrees causes incurable deafness.

Cure. Allay the pain with all convenient speed, but have a care of using strong remedies. Therefore only use warm milk about the ears, with the decoction of poppy tops, or oil of violets: to take away the moisture, use honey of roses, and let aquamollis be dropped into the ears; or take virgin honey half an ounce: red wine, two ounces: allum, saffron, saltpetre, each a dram: mix them at the fire; or drop in hempseed oil with a little wine.

SECTION VI.

Of Redness, and Inflammation of the Buttocks, Groin, and the Thighs of a Young Child.

If there be not great care taken to change and wash the child's bed as soon as it is fouled with the excrements, and to keep the child very clean, the acrimony will be sure to cause redness, and beget a smarting in the buttocks, groin, and thighs of the child, which, by reason of the pain, will afterwards be subject to inflammations, which follow the sooner, through the delicacy and tenderness of their skin, from which the outward skin of the body is in a short time separated and worn away.

Cure. First, keep the child cleanly; and, secondly, take off the sharpness of its urine. As to keeping it cleanly, she must be a sorry nurse that needs to be taught how to do it; for if she lets it have but dry, clean, and warm beds and clouts, as often and as soon as it has fouled and wet them, either by its urine or excrements, it will be sufficient. And as to the taking off the sharpness of the child's urine, that must be done by the nurse's taking a cool diet, that her milk may have the same quality: and therefore she ought to abstain from all things that may tend to heat it.

But besides these, cooling and drying remedies are requisite to be applied to the inflamed parts; therefore let the parts be bathed with plantain-water, with a fourth of lime-water added to it, each time the child's excrements are wiped off; and if the pain be very great, let it only be fomented with luke-warm milk. The powder of a post to dry it, or a little mill-dust strewed upon the parts affected, may be proper enough, and is used by many women. Also, unguentum album, or a diapampoligos, spread upon a small piece of leather, in form of a plaister, will not be amiss.

But the chief thing must be the nurse's taking great care to wrap the inflamed parts with fine rags when she opens the child, that those parts may not gather and be pained by rubbing together.

SECTION VII.

Of Vomiting in Young Children.

Vomiting in children proceeds sometimes from too much milk, and sometimes from bad milk, and as often from a moist loose stomach: for as dryness retains, so looseness lets go. This is, for the most part, without danger in children; and they that vomit from their birth are the lustiest: for the stomach not being used to meat, and milk being taken too much, crudities are easily bred, or the milk is corrupted; and it is better to vomit these up than to keep them in; but if vomiting last long, it will cause an atrophy, or consumption, for want of nourishment.

Cure. If this be from too much milk, that which is emitted is yellow and green, or otherwise ill-coloured and stinking; in this case, mend the milk, as has been showed before cleanse the child with honey of roses, and strengthen its stomach with syrup of milk and quinces made into an electuary. If the humours be hot and sharp, give the syrup of pomegranates, currants, and coral: and apply to the belly the plaister of bread, the stomach cerate, or bread dipped in hot wine: or take oil of mastich, quinces, mint, wormwood, each half an ounce; of nutmegs, by expression half a dram; chymical oil of mint, three drops. Coral hath an occult property to prevent vomiting, and is therefore hung about the neck.

SECTION VIII.

Of Breeding Teeth in young Children.

This is a very great and yet necessary evil in all children, having a variety of symptoms joined with it. They begin to come forth, not all at once, but one after the other, about the sixth or seventh month; the fore-teeth coming first, then the eye-teeth, and, last of all, the grinders. The eye-teeth cause more pain to the child than any of the rest, because they have a deep root, and a small nerve which hath communication with that which makes the eye move.

In the breeding of the teeth, first they feel an itching in their gums, then they are pierced as with a needle, and pricked by the sharp bones, whence proceed great pains, watching, inflammation of the gums, fever, looseness, and convulsions, especially when they breed their eye-teeth.

The signs when children breed their teeth are these:

1. It is known by the time, which is usually about the seventh month.

2. Their gums are swelled, and they feel a great heat there, with an itching, which makes them put their fingers into their mouths to rub them; a moisture also distils from the gums into the mouth, because of the pain they feel there.

3. They hold the nipple faster than before.

4. The gums are white where the teeth begin to come; and the nurse, in giving them such, finds the mouth hotter, and that they are much changed, crying every moment, and cannot sleep, or but very little at a time.

The fever that follows breeding of teeth comes from choleric humours, inflamed by watching, pain, and heat. And the longer teeth are breeding, the more dangerous it is, so that many, in the breeding of them, die of fevers and convulsions.

P

CURE. Two things are to be regarded: one is, to preserve the child from the evil accidents that may happen to it by reason of the great pain; the other, to assist as much as may be the cutting of the teeth, when they can hardly cut the gums themselves.

For the first of these, viz. the preventing these accidents to the child, the nurse ought to take great care to keep a good diet, and to use all things that may cool and temper her milk, that so a fever may not follow the pain of the teeth. And to prevent the humour from falling too much upon the inflamed gums, let the child's belly be kept always loose by gentle clysters, if he be bound: though oftentimes there is no need of them, because they are at those times usually troubled with a looseness; and yet, for all that, clysters may not be improper.

As to the other, which is to assist in cutting the teeth, that the nurse must do from time to time by mollifying and loosening them, and rubbing them with her finger dipped in butter or honey; or let the child have a virgin-wax candle to chew upon; or anoint the gums with the mucilage of quince made with mallow-water, or with the brains of a hare; also foment the cheeks with the decoction of althæa, and camomile flower and dill, or with the juice of mallows and fresh butter. If the gums are inflamed, add juice of nightshade and lettuce. I have already said the nurse ought to take a temperate diet; I shall now only add, that barley-broth, water-gruel, raw eggs, prunes, lettuce and endive, are good for her; but let her avoid salt, sharp, biting, and peppered meats and wine.

SECTION IX.

Of the Flux of the Belly, or Looseness in Infants.

IT is very common for infants to have the flux of the belly, or looseness, especially upon the least indisposition: nor is it to be wondered at, seeing their natural moistness contributes so much thereto: and even if it be extraordinarily violent, such are in a better state of health than those that are bound. The flux, if violent, proceeds from divers causes: as, 1. From breeding of the teeth, and is then commonly attended with a fever, in which the concoction is hindered, and the nourishment corrupted. 2. From watching. 3. From pain. 4. From stirring up of the humours by a fever. 5. When they suck or drink too much in a fever. Sometimes they have a flux without breeding of teeth, from inward cold in the guts or stomach that obstructs concoction. If it be from the teeth, it is easily known; for the signs in breeding of teeth will discover it. If it be from external cold, there are signs of other causes. If from a humour flowing from the head, there are signs of a catarrh, and the excrements are frothy. If crude and raw humours are voided, and there be wind, belching, and phlegmatic excrements: or if they be yellow, green, and stink, the flux is from a hot and sharp humour. It is best in breeding of teeth when the belly is loose, as I have said before: but if it be too violent, and you are afraid it may end in a consumption, it must be stopped; and if the excrements that are voided be black, and attended with a fever, it is very bad.

CURE. The remedy in this case is principally with respect to the nurse, and the condition of the milk must chiefly be observed: the nurse must be cautioned that she eat no green fruit, nor things of hard concoction. If the child suck not, remove the flux with such purges as leave a cooling quality behind them, as syrup of honey or roses, or a clyster. Take the decoction of millium, myrobolans, of each two or three ounces, with an ounce or two of syrup of roses, and make a clyster. After cleansing, if it proceed from a hot cause, give syrup of dried roses, quinces, myrtles, with a little sanguis draconis. Also anoint with oil of roses, myrtles, mastich, each two drams; with oil of myrtles and wax make an ointment. Or take red roses and moulin, of each a handful; cypress roots two drams; make a bag; boil it in red wine, and apply it to the belly. Or, use the plaister of bread, or stomach ointment. If the cause be cold, and the excrements white, give syrup of mastich and quinces, with mint-water. Use outwardly mint, mastich, cummin: or take rose seeds an ounce, cummin, anniseed, each two drams; with oil of mastich, wormwood, and wax make an ointment.

SECTION X.

Of the Epilepsy and Convulsions in Children.

THIS is a distemper that is often fatal to young children, and frequently proceeds from the brain, as when the humours that cause it are bred in the brain, originating either from the parents, or from vapours or bad humours that twitch the membranes of the brain; it is also sometimes caused by other distempers, and by bad diet: likewise the toothach, when the brain consents, causes it, and so does a sudden fright. As to the distemper itself, it is manifest and well enough known where it is; and as to the cause whence it comes, you may know by the signs of the disease, whether it comes from bad milk, or worms, or teeth; if these are all absent, it is certain that the brain is first affected; if it come with the small-pox or measles, it ceaseth when they come forth, if nature be strong enough.

CURE. For the remedy of this grievous and often mortal distemper, give the following powder, to prevent it, to a child, as soon as it is born; take male peony roots, gathered in the decrease of the moon, a scruple; with leaf gold make a powder; or take peony roots a dram; peony seeds, misletoe of the oak, elk's hoof, man's skull, amber, each a scruple; musk, two grains; make a powder. The best part of the cure is taking care of the nurse's diet, which must be regular by all means. If it be from corrupt milk, provoke a vomit; to do which, hold down the tongue, and put a quill, dipped in sweet almonds, down the throat. If it come from the worms, give such things as will kill the worms. If there be a fever, with respect to that also, give coral smaraged and elk's hoof. In the fit, give epileptic water, as lavender water, and rub with oil of amber, or hang a peony root, and elk's hoof smaraged, about the child's neck.

As to a convulsion, it is when the brain labours to cast out that which troubles it; the manner is in the marrow of the back and fountain of the nerves: it is a stubborn disease, and often kills.

Wash the body, when in the fit, especially the back bone, with decoction of althæa, lily roots, peony and camomile flowers, and anoint it with man's and goose's grease, oils of worms, orris, lilies, foxes, turpentine, mastich, storax, and calamint. The sunflower is also very good, boiled in water, to wash the child.

PROPER AND SAFE REMEDIES

FOR CURING ALL THOSE

DISTEMPERS THAT ARE PECULIAR TO

THE FEMALE SEX,

AND

ESPECIALLY THOSE THAT ARE OBSTRUCTIONS TO

BEARING OF CHIDREN.

PART SECOND.

Having finished the first part of this book, and therein, I hope, amply made good my promise to the reader, I am now come to treat of the distempers peculiar to the female sex; in which it is my design to treat only of those to which they are more subject when in a breeding condition, and those that keep them from being so; together with such proper and safe remedies as may be sufficient to repel them. And since, amongst all the diseases to which human nature is subject, there is none which more diametrically opposes the very end of our creation, and the design of nature in the formation of the different sexes, and the power thereby given us for the work of generation, than that of sterility, or barrenness, which, where it prevails, renders the most accomplished midwife but a useless person, and destroys the design of our book; I think, therefore, barrenness is an effect that deserves our first and principal consideration.

CHAPTER I.

Of barrenness; its several Kinds; with the proper Remedies for it; and the Signs of Insufficiency in Men and Women.

SECTION I.

Of Barrenness in general.

BARRENNESS is either natural or artificial.

Natural barrenness is, when a woman is barren though the instruments of generation are perfect both in herself and husband, and no preposterous or diabolical course used to cause it, and neither age nor disease, nor any natural defect hindering, and yet the woman remains naturally barren.

Now this may proceed from a natural cause: for if the man and woman be of one complexion, they seldom have children: and the reason is clear, for the universal course of nature, being formed of a composition of contraries, cannot be increased by a composition of likes; and therefore, if the constitution of the woman be hot and dry, as well as the man, there can be no conception: and if, on the contrary, the man should be of a cold and moist constitution, as well as the woman, the effect would be the same—and this barrenness is purely natural. The only way to help this, is, for people, before they marry, to observe each other's complexion if they design to have children. If their complexions and constitutions be alike, they are not fit to come together, for discordant natures only make harmony in the work of generation.

Another natural cause of barrenness, is want of love between the man and wife. Love is that vital principle that ought to inspire each organ in the act of generation or else it will be spiritless and dull: for if their hearts be not united in love, how should their seed unite to cause conception? And this is sufficiently evinced, in that there never follows conception on a rape. Therefore if men and women design to have children, let them live so that their hearts as well as their bodies may be united, or else they may miss of their expectations.

A third cause of natural barrenness, is the letting virgins blood in the arm before their natural courses are come down, which is usually in the fourteenth and fifteenth years of age—sometimes, perhaps, before the thirteenth, but never before the twelfth. And because usually they are out of order and indisposed before their purgations come down, their parents run to the doctor to know what is the matter: and he, if not skilled, will naturally prescribe opening a vein in the arm, thinking fulness of blood the cause: and thus she seems recovered for the present: and when the young virgin happens to be in the same disorder, the mother applies again to the surgeon, who uses the same remedy: and by these means the blood is so diverted from its proper channel, that it comes not down to the womb as usual: and so the womb dries up, and she is for ever barren. To prevent this, let no virgin blood in the arm before her courses come down well: but, if there be necessity, let her blood in the foot, for that will bring the blood downwards, and by that means provoke the menstrua to come down.

Another cause of natural barrenness is debility in copulation. If persons perform not that act with all the bent and ardour that nature requires, they may as well let it alone, and expect to have children without it; for frigidity and coldness never produce conception. Of the cure of this we will speak by and by, after I have spoken of accidental barrenness, which is occasioned by some morbific matter or infirmity upon the body, either of the man or the woman, which being removed they become fruitful. And since, as I have before noted, the first and great law of the creation was to increase and multiply, and barrenness is in direct opposition to that law, and frustrates the end of our creation: and as it is a great affliction to many to be without children, and often causes man and wife to have hard thoughts one of another: I shall here, for the satisfaction of well-meaning people, set down the signs and causes of insufficiency both in men and women; premising first, that when people have no children, they must not presently blame either party, for neither may be in fault.

SECTION II.

Signs and Causes of Insufficiency in Men.

One cause may be in some viciousness of the yard, as if the same be crooked, or any ligaments thereof distorted and broken, whereby the ways and passages through which the seed should flow come to be stopped or vitiated.

Another cause may be too much weakness of the yard, and tenderness thereof, so that it is not strong enough erected to inject seed into the womb; for the strength and stiffness of the yard very much conduces to conception, by reason of the forcible injection of the seed.

Also, if the stones have received any hurt, so that they cannot exercise the proper gift in producing seed; or if they be oppressed with an inflammation, tumour, wound, or ulcer, or drawn up within the belly, and not appearing outwardly.

Also, a man may be barren by reason of the defect of seed; as, first, if he cast forth no seed at all, or less in substance than is needful. Or, secondly, if the seed be vicious, or unfit for generation; as, on the one side, it happens in bodies that are gross and fat, the matter of it being defective; and, on the other side, too much leanness, or continual wasting or consumption of the body, destroys seed; nature turning all the matter and substance thereof into the nutriment of the body.

Too frequent copulation is also one great cause of barrenness in men; for it attracteth the seminal moisture from the stones, before it is sufficiently prepared and concocted. So if any one, by daily copulation, do exhaust and draw out all the moisture of the seed, then do the stones draw the moist humours from the superior veins into themselves; and so having but little blood in them, they are forced of necessity to cast it out raw and unconcocted, and thus the stones are violently deprived of the moisture of their veins, and the superior veins and all the other parts of the body of their vital spirits; therefore it is no wonder that those who use immoderate copulation are very weak in their bodies, seeing their whole body is therefore deprived of the best and purest blood, and of the spirit, insomuch that many who have been too much addicted to that pleasure, have killed themselves in the very act.

Gluttony, drunkenness, and other excesses, do so much hinder men from fruitfulness, that it makes them unfit for generation.

But among other causes of barrenness among men, this also is one and makes them almost of the nature of eunuchs and that is the incision, or the cutting of their veins behind their ears, which in case of distempers is oftentimes done; for, according to the opinion of most physicians and anatomists, the seed flows from the brain by those veins behind the ears more than from any part of the body. From whence it is very probable, that the transmission of the seed is hindered by the cutting of the veins behind the ears, so that it cannot descend at all to the testicles, or may come thither very crude and raw.

SECTION III.

Signs and Causes of Insufficiency, or Barrenness in Women.

ALTHOUGH there are many causes of the barrenness of women, yet the chief and principal are internal, respecting either the privy parts, the womb, or menstruous blood.

Therefore Hippocrates saith (speaking as well of easy as difficult conceptions in women,) the first consideration is to be had of their species; for little women are more apt to conceive than great, slender than gross, white and fair than ruddy and high coloured, black than wan, those that have their veins conspicuous than others: but to be very fleshy is evil; and to have great swelled breasts is good.

The next thing to be considered, is the monthly purgations, whether they have been duly every month, whether they flow plentifully, are of a good colour, and whether they have been equal every month.

Then the womb, or place of conception, is to be considered. It ought to be clean and sound, dry and soft; not retracted or drawn up; not prone, nor descending downwards; nor the mouth thereof turned away, nor too close shut up. But to speak more particularly:

The first parts to be spoken of are the pudenda, or privities, and the womb: which parts are shut and inclosed, by nature, or against nature; and from hence, such in women are called *impervatores*, as in some women the mouth of their womb continues compressed, or closed up, from the time of their birth until the coming down of their courses, and then, on a sudden, when their terms press forwards to purgation, they are molested with great and unusual pains. Sometimes these break of their own accord; others are dissected and opened by physicians; others never break at all, which bring on disorders that end in death.

All these Aetius particularly handles, showing that the womb is shut three manner of ways, which hinders conception. And the first is, when the lips of the pudenda grow or cleave together. The second is, when there are certain membranes growing in the middle part of the matrix within. The third is, when (though the lips and bosom of the pudenda may appear fair and open) the mouth of the womb may be quite shut up. All which are occasions of barrenness, as they hinder the intercourse with man, the monthly courses, and conception.

But amongst all causes of barrenness in woman, the greatest is in the womb, which is the field of generation: and if this field is corrupt, it is in vain to expect any fruit, let it be ever so well sown. It may be unfit for generation by reason of many distempers to which it is subject: as, for instance, over-much heat, and over much cold; for women whose wombs are too thick and cold cannot conceive because coldness extinguishes the heat of the human seed. Immoderate moisture of the womb also destroys the seed of man, and makes it ineffectual, as corn sown in ponds and marshes; and so does over-much dryness of the womb, so that the seed perisheth for want of nutriment. Immoderate heat of the womb is also a cause of barrenness; for it scorcheth up the seed as corn sown in the drought of summer: for immoderate heat burns all parts of the body, so that no conception can live in the womb.

When unnatural humours are engendered, as too much phlegm, tympanies, wind, water, worms, or any such evil humours abounding contrary to nature, it causes barrenness, as do all terms not coming down in due order.

A woman may also have other accidental causes of barrenness (at least such as may hinder her conception,) as sudden frights, anger, grief, and purterbation of mind; too violent exercises, as leaping, dancing, running after copulation, and the like. But I will now add some signs, by which these things may be known.

If the cause of barrenness be in the man, through overmuch heat in his seed, the woman may easily feel that in receiving it.

If the nature of the woman be too hot, and so unfit for conception, it will appear by having her terms very little, and the colour inclining to yellowness, she is also very hasty, choleric, and crafty; her pulse beats very swift, and she is very desirous of copulation.

To know whether the fault is in the man or in the woman, sprinkle the man's urine upon a lettuce leaf, and the woman's urine upon another, and that which dries away first is unfruitful. Also take five wheaten corns and seven beans, put them into an earthen pot, and let the party make water therein; let this stand seven days, and if in that time they begin to sprout, then the party is fruitful; but if they sprout not, then the party is barren, whether it be man or woman: this is a certain sign.

There are some that make this experiment of a woman's fruitfulness: take myrrh, red storax, and some odoriferous things, and make a perfume of it; which let the woman receive into the neck of the womb through a funnel; if the woman feels the smoke ascend through her body to the nose, then she is fruitful, otherwise she is barren. Some also take garlic and beer, and cause the woman to lie on her back upon it, and if she feel the scent thereof in her nose, it is a sign of her being fruitful.

Culpepper and others also give a great deal of credit to the following experiment: take a handful of barley, and steep half of it in the urine of the man, and the other half in the urine of the woman, for the space of twenty-four hours; then take it out, and put the man's by itself, and the woman's by itself; set it in a flower pot, or some other thing, where let it dry; water the man's every morning with his own urine, and the woman's with hers, and that which grows first is the most fruitful; but if they grow not at all, they are both naturally barren.

CURE. If barrenness proceed from stoppage of the menstrua, let the woman sweat, for that opens the parts: and the best way to sweat is in a hot-house. Then let the womb be strengthened by drinking a draught of white wine, wherein a handful of stinking arrack, first bruised, has been boiled; for by a secret magnetic virtue it strengthens the womb, and by a simpathetic quality, removes any disease thereof. To which add also a handful of vervain, which is very good to strengthen both the womb and the head, which are commonly afflicted together by sympathy. Having used these two or three days, if they come not down, take of calamint, pennyroyal, thyme, betony, bittany, burnet, feverfew, mugwort, sage, peony roots, juniper berries, half a handful of each, or so many as can be got; let these be boiled in beer, and taken for her drink.

Take one part of gentian-root, two parts of cantaury, distil them with ale in an alembic, after you have bruised the gentian roots, and infused them well. This water is an admirable remedy to provoke the terms. But if you have not this water in readiness, take a dram of centory, and half a dram of gentian root bruised, boiled in posset drink, and drink a draught of it at night going to bed. Seed of wild navew beaten to powder, and a dram of it taken in the morning in white wine, also is very good; but if it answer not, she must be let blood in the legs. And be sure you administer your medicines a little before the full of the moon, or before the new and full moon, by no means in the wane of the moon, if you do, you will find them ineffectual.

If barrenness proceed from the overflowing of the menstrua, then strengthen the womb as you were taught before; afterwards anoint the reins of the back with oil of roses, oil of myrtle, oil of quinces, every night, and then wrap a piece of white baize about your reins, the cotton side next the skin, and keep the same always to it. But, above all, I recommend this medicine to you. Take comfrey leaves or roots, and clown wound-wort, of each a handful; bruise them well, and boil them in ale, and drink a good draught of it now and then. Or take cinnamon, cassia lignea, opium, of each two drams, myrrh, white pepper, galbanum, of each one dram; dissolve the gum and opium in white wine: beat the rest into powder, and make it into pills, mixing them together exactly, and let the patient take two every night going to bed; but let the pills not exceed fifteen grains.

If barrenness proceed from a flux in the womb, the cure must be according to the cause producing it, or which the flux proceeds from, which may be known by signs: for a flux of the womb, being a continual distillation from it for a long time together, the colour of what is voided shows what humour it is that offends; in some it is red, and that proceeds from blood putrified; in some it is yellow, and that denotes choler; in others white and pale, and that denotes phlegm. If pure blood comes out, as if a vein were opened, some corrosion or gnawing of the womb is to be feared. All these are known by the following signs.

The place of conception is continually moist with the humours, the face is ill-coloured, the party loathes meat, and breathes with difficulty, the eyes are much swollen, which is sometimes without pain. If the offending humour be pure blood, then you must let blood in the arm, and the cephalic vein is fittest to draw back the blood: then let the juice of plantain and comfrey be injected into the womb. If phlegm be the cause, let cinnamon be a spice used in all her meats and drinks; and let her take a little Venice treacle or mithridate every morning. Let her boil burnet, mugwort, feverfew, and vervain, in all her broths. Also, half a dram of myrrh, taken every morning, is an excellent remedy against this malady. If choler be the cause, let her take buriage, buglos, red roses, endive, and succory-roots, lettuce and white poppy seed, of each a handful; boil these in white wine till one half be wasted; let her drink half a pint every morning; to which half a pint add syrup of peach flowers and syrup of chicony, of each an ounce, with a little rhubarb, and this will gently purge her. If it proceed from putrified blood, let her be bled in the foot then strengthen the womb as I have directed in stopping of the menstrua.

If barrenness be occasioned by the falling out of the womb as sometimes it happens, let her apply sweet scents to the nose, such as civet, galbanum, storax, calamitis, wood of aloes, and such other things as are of that nature; and let her lay stinking things to the womb, such as assafœtida, oil of amber, or the smoke of her own hair, being burnt; for this is a certain truth, that the womb flies from all stinking, and to all sweet things. But the most infallible cure, in this case is: take a common burdoc-leaf (which you may keep dry, if you please, all the year,) apply this to her head, and it will draw the womb upwards. In fits of the mother, apply it to the soles of her feet, and it will draw the womb downwards. But seed beaten in a powder, draws the womb which way you please, according as it is applied.

If barrenness in the woman proceed from a hot cause, let her take whey, and clarify it; then boil plantain-leaves and roots in it, and drink it for her ordinary drink. Let her also inject the juice of plantain into her womb with a syringe. If it be winter, when you cannot get the juice, make a strong decoction of the leaves and roots in water, and inject that up with a syringe; but let it be blood warm, and you will find this medicine of great efficacy. And further, to take away barrenness proceeding from hot causes: take of conserve of roses, cold lozenges made of tragacanth, the confections of tricantelia; and use, to smell to, camphire, rose water, and saunders. It is also good to bleed the basilica, or liver-vein, and take four or five ounces of blood, and then take this purge: take electuarium de epithymo, de succo rosarum, of each two drams and a half; clarified whey, four ounces: mix them well together, and take it in the morning fasting: sleep after it about an hour and a half, and fast four hours after; and about an hour before you eat any thing, drink a good draught of whey. Also take lily-water, four ounces; mandragar water, one ounce; saffron half a scruple; beat the saffron to powder, and mix it with the waters, drink them warm in the morning; use them eight days together.

Q

Some approved Remedies against Barrenness, and to cause Fruitfulness.

Take broom flowers, smallage, parsley seed, cummin, mugwort, feverfew, of each half a scruple; aloes, half an ounce; Indian salt, saffron, of each half a dram; beat and mix them together, and put to it five ounces of feverfew water warm, stop it close up, and let it stand and dry in a warm place, and this do two or three times, one after another; then make each dram into six pills, and take one of them every other night before supper.

For purging medicine against barrenness take conserve of benedicta lax, a quarter of an ounce; depsillo, three drams; electuary de succo rosarum, one dram; mix them together with feverfew water, and drink it in the morning betimes.— About three days after the patient hath taken the purge, let her be bled, taking four or five ounces in the midian, or common black vein in the right foot; and then give for five successive days, filed ivory, a dram and a half, in feverfew water; and during the time let her sit in the following bath an hour together, morning and night. Take mild yellow saps, daucus, balsam wood and fruit, ashkeys, of each two handfuls, red and white behen, broom flowers, of each a handful: musk, three grains; amber, saffron, of each a scruple; boil all in water sufficiently; but the musk, saffron, amber, and broom flowers must be put into the decoction, after it is boiled and strained.

A Confection very good against Barrenness.

Take pistachia, eringoes, of each half an ounce; saffron, one dram; lignum aloes, galingal, mace, coriophille, balm flowers, red and white behen, of each four scruples; ivory shavings, cassia bark, of each two scruples: syrup of confected ginger, twelve ounces: white sugar six ounces: decoct all these in twelve ounces of balm water, and stir them well together: then put to it musk and amber, of each a scruple: take thereof the quantity of a nutmeg three times a day: in the morning, an hour before noon, and an hour after supper.

But if the cause of barrenness, either in man or woman, be through scarcity of diminution of the natural seed, then such things are to be taken as do increase the seed, and incite or stir up to venery and further conception: which I shall here set down, and then conclude this chapter concerning barrenness.

For this, yellow rape seed baked in bread is very good; also young fat flesh, not too much salted; also saffron, the tails of stincus, and long pepper prepared in wine. But let such persons eschew all sour, sharp, doughy and slimy meats, long sleep after meat, surfeiting, and drunkenness; and so much as they can, keep themselves from sorrow, grief, vexation, and anxious care.

These things following increase the natural seed, stir up venery, and recover the seed again when it is lost, viz. eggs, milk, rice boiled in milk, sparrows' brains, flesh, bones and all: the stones and pizzles of bulls, bucks, rams, and bears; also cocks' stones, lambs' stones, partridges, quails, and pheasants' eggs. And this is an undeniable aphorism, that whatever any creature is addicted unto, they move or incite the man or woman that eats them to the like; and therefore partridges, quails, sparrows, &c. being extremely addicted to venery, they work the same effect on those men and women that eat them. Also take notice, that in what part of the body the faculty which you would strengthen lies, take the same part of the body of another creature, in whom the faculty is strong, as a medicine. As for instance, the procreative faculty lies in the testicles; therefore cocks' stones, lambs' stones, &c. are proper to stir up venery. I will also give you another general rule: all creatures that are fruitful being eaten makes them fruitful that eat them, as crabs, lobsters, prawns, pigeons, &c. The stones of a fox dried and beaten to powder, and a dram taken in the morning in sheep's milk, and the stones of a boar taken in like manner, are very good. The heart of a male quail carried about the man, and the heart of a female quail carried about the woman, causeth natural love and fruitfulness. Let them also that would increase their seed eat and drink of the best as much as they can: for *sine cerere et libero friget Venus* is an old proverb: which is, " Without good meat and drink, Venus will be frozen to death.

Pottages are good to increase the seed; such as are made of beans, peas, and lupines, mixed with sugar, French beans, wheat sodden in broth, anniseed, also onions stewed, garlic, leeks, yellow rapes, fresh mugwort roots, eringo roots confected, ginger confected, &c. Of fruits, hazel nuts, cyprus nuts, pistachia, almonds, and marchpanes thereof, Spices good to increase seed are cinnamon, galengal, long pepper, cloves, ginger, saffron, assafœtida; a dram and a half taken in good wine, is very good for this purpose.

The weakness and debility of a man's yard being a great hinderance to procreation, let him use the following ointment to strengthen it: take wax, oil of beaver, cod, marjoram gentle, and oil of coflus, of each a like quantity, mix them into an ointment, and put to it a little musk, and with it anoint the yard, cods, &c. Take of house emmets three drams, oil of white saffanum, oil of lilies, of each an ounce; pound and bruise the ants, and put them to the oil, and let them stand in the sun six days: then strain out the oil, and add to it euphorbium one scruple, pepper and rue, of each one dram; mustard seed half a dram; set this altogether in the sun two or three days, then anoint the instrument of generation therewith.

CHAPTER II.

The Diseases of the Womb.

I HAVE already said, that the womb is the field of generation; and if this field be corrupted, it is in vain to expect any fruit, though it be ever so well sown. It is therefore not without reason that I intend in this chapter to set down the several distempers to which the womb is obnoxious, with proper and safe remedies against them.

SECTION I.

Of the hot Distempers of the Womb.

THIS distemper consists in excess of heat: for as heat of the womb is necessary for conception, so if it be too much, it nourisheth not the seed, but disperseth its heat, and hinders the conception. This preternatural heat is sometimes from the birth, and causes barrenness; but if it be accidental, it is from hot causes, that bring the heat and the blood to the womb; it arises also from internal and external medicines, and from too much hot meat, drink, or exercise. Those that are troubled with this distemper have but few courses, and those are yellow, black, burnt, or sharp: have hair betimes on their privities; are very prone to lust, subject to the headach, and abound with choler; and when the distemper is strong upon them, they have but few terms, which are out of order, being bad and hard to flow, and in time they become hypochondriacs, and for the most part barren, having sometimes a frenzy of the womb.

CURE. The remedy is to use coolers, so that they offend not the vessels that must be open for the flux of the terms,

Therefore, take inwardly, succory, endive, violets, water lilies, sorrel, lettuce, saunders, and syrups and conserves made thereof. Also take conserve of succory, violets, water lilies, burrage, each an ounce; conserve of roses, half an ounce; diamargation frigid, diatriascantal, each half a dram; and with syrup of violets, or juice of citrons, make an electuary. For outward applications, make use of ointment of roses, violets, water lilies, gourd, venus navel, applied to the back and loins.

Let the air be cool, her garments thin, and her food endive, lettuce, succory, and barley. Give her no hot meats, nor strong wine, unless mixed with water. Rest is good for her; but she must abstain from copulation, though she may sleep as long as she pleases.

SECTION II.

Of the Cold Distemper of the Womb.

THIS distemper is the reverse of the foregoing, and equally an enemy to generation, being caused by a cold quality abounding to excess, and proceeds from a too cold air, rest, idleness, and cooling medicines. It may be known by an aversion to venery, and taking no pleasure in the act of copulation when the seed is spent; the terms are phlegmatic, thick, and slimy, and do not flow as they should; the womb is windy, and the seed crude and waterish. It is the cause of obstructions and barrenness, and hard to be cured.

CURE. Take galengal, cinnamon, nutmeg, mace, cloves, each two drams; ginger, cubebs, zedoary, cardamum, each an ounce; grains of paradise, long pepper, each half an ounce; beat them, and put them into six quarts of wine for eight days: then add sage, mint, balm, motherwort, of each three handsful: let them stand eight days more; then poor off the wine, and beat the herbs and the spice, and then pour on the wine again, and distil them. Or you may use this: take cinnamon, nutmeg, cloves, mace, ginger, cubebs, cardamum, grains of paradise, each an ounce and a half; galengal six drams, long pepper half an ounce, zedoary five drams; bruise them, and add six quarts of wine; put them into a cellar nine days, daily stirring them: then add of mint two handsful, and let them stand fourteen days: pour off the wine, and bruise them, and then pour on the wine again, and distil them. Also anoint with oil of lilies, rue, angelica, bays, cinnamon, cloves, mace and nutmeg. Let her diet and air be warm, her meat of easy concoction, seasoned with anniseed, fennel, and thyme: and let her avoid raw fruits and milk diets.

SECTION III.

Of the Inflation of the Womb.

THE inflation of the womb is a stretching of it by wind, called by some a windy mole; the wind proceeds from a cold matter, whether thick or thin, contained in the veins of the womb, by which the weak heat thereof is overcome, and which either flows thither from other parts, or is gathered there by cold meats and drinks. Cold air may be the producing cause of it also, as women that lie in are exposed to it. The wind is contained either in the cavity of the vessels of the womb, or between the tunicles, and may be known by a swelling in the region of the womb, which sometimes reaches to the navel, loins, and diaphragm, and rises and abates as the wind increaseth or decreaseth. It differs from the dropsy, in that it never swells so high. That neither physician nor midwife may take it for a conception, let them observe the signs of the women with child, laid down in a former part of this work; and if any sign be wanting, they may suspect it to be an inflation; of which this is a further sign, that in conception the swelling is variable; also, if you strike upon the belly, in an inflation, there will be a noise, but not so in case there be a conception. It also differs from a mole, because in that there is a weight and hardness in the belly, and when the patient moves from one side to the other she feels a great weight which moveth; but not so in this. If the inflation continue without the cavity of the womb, the pain is greater and more extensive, nor is there any noise, because the wind is more pent up.

CURE. This distemper is neither of a long continuance, nor dangerous, if looked after in time; and if it be in the cavity of the womb, is more easily expelled. To which purpose give her diaphnicon, with a little castor, and sharp clysters that expel wind. If this distemper happen to a woman in travail, let her not purge after delivery, nor bleed, because it is from a cold matter; but if it come after child bearing, and her terms come down sufficiently, and she has fulness of blood, let the sapæna vein be opened; after which, let her take the following electuary: take conserve of betony and rosemary, of each an ounce and a half; candied eringoes, citron peel candied, each half an ounce; diacimium, diagalangal, each a dram; oil of anniseed six drops; and with syrup of citrons make an electuary. For outward application make a cataplasm of rue, mugwort, camomile, dill, calamint, new pennyroyal, thyme, with oil of rue, keir, and camomile. And let the following clyster, to expel wind, be put into the womb: take agnus, castus, cinnamon, each two drams, boil them in wine to half a pint. She may likewise use sulphur, Bath and Spa waters, both inward and outward because they expel wind.

SECTION IV.

Of the Straitness of the Womb, and its Vessels.

This is another effect of the womb, which is a very great obstruction to the bearing of children, hindering both the flow of the menses and conception, and is seated in the vessels of the womb, and the neck thereof. The causes of this straitness are thick and rough humours, that stop the mouths of the veins and arteries. These humours are bred either by gross or too much nourishment, when the heat of the womb is so weak that it cannot attenuate the humours, which, by reason thereof, either flow from the whole body, or are gathered into the womb. Now, the vessels are made straiter or closer several ways: sometimes by inflammation, schirrous, or other tumours; sometimes by compressions, scars, or by flesh or membranes that grow after a wound. The signs by which this is known are, the stoppage of the terms, not conceiving, and crudities abounding in the body, which are all shown by particular signs; for if there is a wound, or the secundine pulled out by force, phlegm comes from the wound; if stoppage of the terms be from an old obstruction by humours, it is hard to be cured; if it be only from the disorderly use of astringents, it is more curable; if it be from a schirrous, or other tumours, that compress or close the vessel, the disease is incurable.

Cure. For the cure of that which is curable, obstructions must be taken away, phlegm must be purged, and she must be let blood, as will be hereafter directed in the stoppage of the terms. Then use the following medicines: take of anniseed and fennel seed, each a dram; rosemary, pennyroyal, calamint, betony flowers, each an ounce; castus, cinnamon, galengal, each half an ounce: saffron, half a dram, with wine. Or take asparagus roots, parsley roots, each an ounce; pennyroyal, calamint, each a handful; wall-flowers, gilly flowers each two handsful; boil, strain, and add syrup of mugwort, an ounce and a half. For a fomentation, take pennyroyal, mercury, calamint, marjoram, mugwort, each two handsful: sage, rosemary, bays, camomile flowers, each a handful; boil them in water, and foment the groin and bottom of the belly; or let her sit up to the navel in a bath, and then anoint about the groin with oil of rue, lilies, dill, &c.

SECTION V.

Of the Falling of the Womb.

This is another evil effect of the womb, which is both very troublesome, and also a hinderance to conception. Sometimes the womb falleth to the middle of the thighs, nay, almost to the knees, and may be known then by its hanging out. Now, that which causeth the womb to change its place is, that the ligaments, by which it is bound to the other parts, are not in order; for there are four ligaments, two above, broad and membraneous, that come from the peritoneum, and two below, that are nervous, round and hollow; it is also bound to the great vessels by veins and arteries, and to the back by nerves; but the place is changed when it is drawn another way, or when the ligaments are loose, and it falls down by its own weight. It is drawn on one side when the menses are hindered from flowing; and the veins and arteries are full, namely, those that go to the womb. If it be a mole on one side, the liver and spleen cause it; by the liver veins on the right side, and the spleen on the left, as they are more or less filled. Others are of opinion, it comes from the solution of the connection of the fibrous neck and the parts adjacent; and that it is from the weight of the womb descending: this we deny not; but the ligaments must be loose or broken. But women in a dropsy could not be said to have the womb fallen down, if it came only from looseness: but in them it is caused by the saltness of the water, which dries more than it moistens. Now, if there be a little tumour, within or without the privities, like a skin stretched, or a weight felt upon the privities, it is nothing else but a descent of the womb; but if there be a tumour like a goose egg, and a hole at the bottom, and there is at first a great pain in the parts to which the womb is fastened, as the loins, the bottom of the belly, and the os sacrum, it proceeds from the breaking or stretching of the ligaments: and a little after, the pain is abated, and there is an impediment in walking, and sometimes blood comes from the breach of the vessels, and the excrements and urine are stopped, and then a fever and convulsion ensueth, oftentimes proving mortal, especially if it happen to women with child.

Cure. For the cure of this distemper, first put up the womb before the air alter it or it be swollen or inflamed; and for this purpose give a clyster to remove the excrements, and then lay her upon her back, with her legs abroad, and her thighs lifted up, and head down; then take the tumour in your hand, and thrust it in without violence; if it be swelled by alteration and cold, foment it with the decoction of mallows, althæa, lime fenugreek, camomile flowers, bay berries, and anoint it with oil of lilies, and hen's grease. If there be an inflammation, do not put it up, but fright it in, by putting a red hot iron before it, and making a show as if you intended to burn it; but first sprinkle upon it the powder of mastich frankincense, and the like: thus, take frankincense, mastich, each two drams; sarcocol, steeped in milk, a dram; mummy, pomegranate flowers, sanguis draconis, each half a dram. When it is put up, let her lie with her legs stretched and one upon the other, for eight or ten days; and make a pessary in the form of a pear, with cork or spunge, and put it into the womb, dipped in sharp wine or juice of acasia, with powder of sanguis with galbanum and bdellium. Also apply a cupping glass, with a great flame, under the navel or paps, or to both kidneys, and lay this plaister to the back: take opoponax two ounces; storax liquid, half an ounce; mastich, frankincense, pitch, bole, each two drams; then with wax make s plaister: or, take laudanum, a dram and a half; mastich, and frankincense, each half a dram; wood aloes, cloves, spike, each a dram; and coloured ambergris, four grains; musk half a scruple; make two round plaisters to be laid on each side of the navel; make a fume of snails' skins salted, or of garlic, and let it be taken in by the funnel. Use also astringent fomentations of bramble leaves, plantain, horse tails, myrtles each two handfuls; wormseed two handfuls; pomegranate flowers half an ounce; boil them in wine and water. For an injection take comfrey roots an ounce; rapture wort, two drams; yarrow, mugwort, each half an ounce; boil them in red wine, and inject it with a syringe. To strengthen the womb take hartshorn, bays, of each a dram; myrrh, half a dram; make a powder for two doses, and give it with sharp wine. Or, you may take zedoary, parsnip seed, crabs' eyes prepared, each a dram; nutmeg half a dram; and give a dram in powder; but astringents must be used with great caution, lest by stopping the courses a worse mischief follow. To keep it in its place, make rollers and ligatures as for rupture; and put pessaries into the bottom of the womb, that may force it to remain. Let the diet be such as has drying, astringent, and glewing qualities, as rice, starch, quinces, pears, and green cheese; but let summer fruits be avoided; and let her wine be astringent and red.

CHAPTER III.

Of Diseases relating to Women's Monthly Courses.

SECTION I.

Of Women's Monthly Courses in General.

THAT Divine Providence, which, with a wisdom peculiar to itself, has appointed woman to conceive by coition with man, and to bear and bring forth children, has provided for the nourishment of children during their recess in the womb of their mother by that redundancy of the blood which is natural to all women, and which, flowing out at certain periods of time (when they are not pregnant,) are from thence called *terms* and *menses*, from their monthly flux of excrementitious blood. Now, that the matter flowing forth its excrementitious, is to be understood only with respect to the redundancy and overplus thereof, being an excrement only with respect to its quantity; for as to its quality, it is as pure and incorrupt as any blood in the veins; and this appears from the final cause of it, which is the propagation and conservation of mankind; and also from the generation of it, being the superfluity of the last aliment of the fleshy parts. If any ask, if the menses be not of a hurtful quality, how can they cause such venemous effects; if they fall upon trees and herbs, they make the one barren, and mortify the other? I answer, this malignity is contracted in the womb; for the woman wanting native heat to digest the superfluity, sends it to the matrix, where seating itself till the mouth of the womb be dilated, it becomes corrupt and mortified; which may easily be, considering the heat and moistness of the place; and so this blood being out of its proper vessels, and too long retained, offends in quality,

SECTION II.

Of Terms coming out of Order, either before or after the usual time.

HAVING in the former part of this work treated of the suppression and overflowing of the monthly terms, I shall content myself with referring the reader thereto, and proceed to speak of their coming out of order, either before or after the usual time.

Both those proceed from an ill constitution of body. Every thing is beautiful in its order, in nature as well as in morality; and if the order of nature be broke, it shows the body to be out of order. Of each of these effects briefly:

When the monthly courses come before their time, showing a depraved excretion, and flowing sometimes twice a month, the cause is in the blood, which stirs up the expulsive faculty in the womb, or else in the whole body, and is frequently occasioned by the person's diet, which increases the blood too much, making it too sharp or too hot. If the retentive faculty of the womb be weak, and the expulsive faculty strong, and of a quick sense, it brings them forth the sooner. Sometimes they flow sooner by reason of a fall, stroke, or some violent passion, which the parties themselves can best relate. If it be from heat, thin and sharp humours, it is known by the distemper of the whole body. The looseness of the vessels, and weakness of the retentive faculty is known from a moist and loose habit of the body. It is more troublesome than dangerous, but hinders conception, and therefore the cure is necessary for all, but especially such as desire children. If it proceed from a sharp blood, let her temper it by a good diet and medicines. To which purpose let her use baths of iron water, that correct the distemper or the bowels, and then evacuate. If it proceed from the retentive faculty, and looseness of the vessels, it is to be corrected with gentle astringents.

As to the courses flowing after the usual time, the causes are, thickness of the blood, and the smallness of its quantity, with the straitness of the passage, and weakness of the expulsive faculties. Either of these singly may stop the courses, but if they all concur, they render the distemper the worse. If the blood abounds not in such a quantity as may stir up nature to expel it, its purging must necessarily be deferred till there be enough. And if the blood be thick, the passage stopped, and the expulsive faculty weak, the menses must needs be out of order, and the purging of them retarded.

For the cure of this, if the quantity of blood be small, let her use a larger diet, and very little exercise. If the blood be thick and foul, let it be made thin, and the humours mixed therewith be evacuated. It is good to purge after the courses have done flowing, and to use calamint; and indeed the oftener she purges the better. She may also use fumes and pessaries, apply cupping glasses without scarification to the inside of the thighs, and rub the legs, and scarify the ancles, and hold the feet in warm water four or five days before the courses come down. Let her also anoint the bottom of her belly with things proper to provoke the terms.

Remedies for disorders in Women's Paps.

Make a cataplasm of bean meal and salad oil, and lay it to the place afflicted. Or anoint with the juice of papilaris. This must be done when the paps are very sore.

If the paps be hard and swelled, take a handful of rue, colewort roots, horehound and mint; if you cannot get all these conveniently, any two will do; pound the handful in honey, and apply it once every day till healed.

If the nipples be stiff and sore, anoint twice a day with Florence oil till healed.

If the paps be flabby and hanging, bruise a little hemlock, and apply it to the breast for three days; but let it not stand above seven hours. Or, which is safer, rusæ juice well boiled, with a little smapios added thereunto, and anoint.

If the paps be hard and dead, make a plate of lead, pretty thin, to answer the breasts: let this stand nine hours each day, for three days. Or, sassafras bruised and used in like manner.

Recipe for procuring Milk.

Drink arpleni, drawn as tea, for 21 days. Or, eat often anniseeds. Also, the juice of arbor vitæ, a glass-ful once a day for eleven days, is very good, for it quickens the memory, strengthens the body, and causeth milk to flow in abundance.

Directions for Drawing of Blood.

Drawing of blood was at first invented for good and salutary purposes, although often abused and misapplied.

To bleed in the left arm removes long continued pain and headachs. It is also good for those who have got falls and bruises.

Bleeding is good for many disorders, and generally proves a cure, except in some very extraordinary cases; and in those cases bleeding is hurtful.

If a woman be pregnant, to draw a little blood will give her ease, good health and a lusty child.

Bleeding is a most certain cure for no less than twenty-one disorders, without any outward or inward applications: and for many more, with application of drugs, herbs, and flowers.

When the moon is on the increase, you may let blood at any time, day or night; but when she is on the decline, you must bleed only in the morning.

Bleeding may be performed from the month of March to November. No bleeding in December, January, or February, unless an occasion requires it. The months of March, April, and November are the three chief months of the year for bleeding in: but it may be performed with safety from the 9th of March to the 19th of November.

To prevent the dangers that may arise from the unskilful drawing of blood, let none open a vein but a person of experience and practice. There are three sorts of people you must not let draw blood; first, ignorant and inexperienced pretenders. Secondly, those who have bad sight and trembling hands, whether skilled or unskilled. For when the hand trembles, the lance is apt to startle from the vein, and the flesh be thereby damaged, which may hurt, canker, and very much torment the patient. Thirdly, let no women bleed you, but such as has gone through a course of midwifery at college: for those who are unskilful may cut an artery, to the great damage of the patient. Besides, what is still worse, those pretended bleeders who take it up at their own hand generally keep unedged and rusty lancets, which will prove hurtful even in a skilful hand. Accordingly, you ought to be cautious in choosing your physician: a man of learning knows what vein to open for each disorder; he knows how much blood to take as soon as he sees the patient; and he can give you suitable advice concerning your disorder.

R

ARISTOTLE'S
LAST LEGACY;

FULLY UNFOLDING

THE MYSTERIES OF NATURE IN THE GENERATION OF MAN.

INTRODUCTION.

WHEN the Almighty Architect of the world had formed the heavens in the beginning, and laid the foundations of the earth, and had created a fair and beautiful world out of a rude mass and undigested chaos, and by his powerful fiat had brought into being all the several species of vegetables and animals, and given even to the plants and vegetables to have seed in themselves for producing their several kinds of form, and to the animals (which he created male and female) the power of propagating their species, and had adorned the world with all these beautiful and glorious embellishments that his consummate wisdom and goodness saw fit and requisite for the wonderful guest he designed to bring into it, he at last created man, as a microcosm or lesser world, to be lord of this greater world, not with a bare fiat only, as he did the rest of his creatures, but called as it were a council of the sacred Trinity about it, saying, " Let US make man in our own image, after our own likeness," &c. as the divine historian expresses: so that man, in his original, is a ray of the Divinity, and the very breath of the Almigthy; and therefore it is said, " God breathed into his nostrils the breath of life, and he became a living soul." Man being thus created, and made lord of the world, had in himself at first both sexes; for the text tells us, " Male and female created he them, and called their name Adam." But yet still Adam was divided, he was still alone: though every other living creature had a mate, he had none, though he was lord of all; so that in Paradise itself, he seemed to be unhappy, wanting a meet help; and therefore his munificent Maker, resolving to make him completely happy, divides him from himself, that by a more agreeable conjunction he might be united to himself again; and so of a part of himself was formed Eve, whom Adam having never seen before, by sympathy of nature presently called "bone of his bone, and flesh of his flesh." And Adam having thus found an help mate given him by his Creator, he became now completely happy; and being blessed by the Almighty, had this law also given him, to increase and multiply, he being endowed with a natural propension thereunto, and the woman having a plastic power given her by nature for the formation of the embryo. This natural inclination and propension of the sexes to each other, with the plastic power of nature, is only the energy of the first blessing and command of the Almighty, and which, to this day, upholds the world

The mystery of the generation of that noblest piece of creation, man, and the unfolding of that plastic power of nature in the secret workings, of generation, and formation of the seed in the womb, was the subject of the foregoing treatise; a subject so necessary to be known by all the female sex (the conception and bearing of children being that which nature has ordained their province) that many, for want of the knowledge, perish, with the fruit of their womb also, who, had they but understood the secret of generation displayed in that book, might have been still in the land of the living.

It is therefore for the use of such that this and the preceding treatises were compiled; wherein the mystery of generation is not only unravelled, and the abstruce secrets of nature made known, but the obstructions and hindrances of generation are declared, and proper remedies against all the defects of the womb most fully prescribed.

CHAPTER I.

Of Virginity, what it is, its Signs and Tokens, and how a Man may know whether he marries a Virgin or not.

THE great Maker of the Universe, who gives all creatures life and being, and a power in themselves to propagate their kind or species, even to the end of the world, has to that end created them male and female: and these two of contrary natures and qualities; for in this noble pair, viz. man and woman, the man is hot and dry, the woman cold and moist; and these two different qualities uniting are ordained by nature for the procreation of children, the seed of the man being the efficient cause, and the womb of the woman the field of generation, wherein the seed is nourished, and the embryo conceived and formed, and in due time brought forth.

Since the woman then has so great a part in the generation of man, I shall endeavour to show how nature has fitted her for it; and because a knowledge of the disease (be it what it will) is half the cure, I have already, in a foregoing part of this work, given a full description of the several parts or members of generation; that so, at any time, if any part be affected or out of order, it may be sooner rectified.

And since the first state of woman is virginity; in speaking of it I will first show what it is, and then lay down some signs and tokens of it, by which it may be known.

Virginity is the boast and pride of the fair sex, though they generally commend it to put it off, and that they may the sooner get a good husband, and thereby lose it: and I think they are in the right of it: for if they keep it too long it grows useless, or at least abates much of its value: a stale virgin (if such a thing there be) being looked upon like an old almanac, out of date. Virginity is the chief, the best, the prime of any thing, and is properly the integrity of a woman's privities, not violated by man, nor known by him, it being the property of a virgin not to have known a man. But to come a little more close, there is in the neck of the womb of young maids a pendulous production, called the *hymen*, which is like the bud of a rose half blown, and this is broken in the first act of copulation with a man, and from thence came the word *defloro*, or deflower, because the taking away of virginity is deflowering a virgin; for, when this rose-bud is expanded, virginity is wholly lost.

Certain it is, there is in the first act of copulation something that causeth pain and bleeding, which is an evident sign of virginity; but what it is, authors agree not; some say it is a nervous membrane, or thin skin, with small veins, which bleeds at the first penetration of the yard; others say, it is four carbuncles, or bits of flesh, or little buds, like myrtle-berries, and these are plump and full in virgins, but hang loose and flag in those who have used carnal copulation, being pressed by the yard; some have observed a fleshy circle about the *nymphæ*, or neck of the womb, with little obscure veins, which make the membrane not to be nervous but fleshy.

There is no doubt but that the part which receiveth the yard is not in women that have used a man, as it is in virgins; and yet it is not alike in all, which have caused that diversity of opinions both among authors and anatomists, for this is not found in all virgins. Excess of lust, or desire of a man, in some, may break the hymen, or *claustrum virginale.* Sometimes, when it itcheth, they put in their finger, and so break it; and sometimes the midwives break it in the birth. Sometimes it is done by stopping of the urine, coughing, violence, straining, or sneezing: and therefore, if there be no bleeding at the first penetration, it is not always a sign of unchastity; but where there is bleeding, it is an unquestionable proof of virginity.

Leo Africanus makes mention of a custom of the Africans at their weddings, which was this: After they were married, the bridegroom and the bride were shut up in a chamber, while the wedding dinner was preparing: and an old woman stood at the chamber door to receive from the bridegroom a sheet having the bloody tokens of the wife's virginity, which she showed in triumph to all the guests, and then they feasted altogether with joy: but if there was no blood to be seen, the bride was sent home to her friends with disgrace, and the disappointed guests went sadly home without their dinner. But notwithstanding the African custom, I affirm, that some honest virgins have lost their maidenheads without bleeding, and therefore are not to be censured, as many ignorant men do, who, for want of this token, cause their wives to lead an uncomfortable life all their days: those coxcombs (though not cuckolds) fancying themselves to have horns on their heads when it is not so.

Some make the straitness of the privities to be a sign of virginity, but this is no certain rule: for much depends upon the age, habit of body, and other circumstances: though it cannot but be acknowledged, that women who have used carnal copulation are not so strait as virgins, yet this can be no certain argument of virginity for after repeated acts of venery, the privities may be made so strait by the use of astringent medicines, that a whore may be sometimes taken for a virgin: and Culpepper mentions a woman that was married, who, desirous to appear a virgin, used a bath of comfrey roots, whereby she deceived those who had to do with her.

Some there are who make milk in the breasts a sign of lost virginity, not considering that there is a twofold milk, the one of virgins being a malady contrary to nature, the other natural: the first is made of blood that cannot get out of the womb, and so goes to the breasts, being nothing but a superfluous nourishment that is turned into milk by the faculty of the breasts, without knowledge of a man: the other is only when there is a child either in the womb, or born: yet the milk differs very much, both in respect of the blood and diversity of veins that bring it to the breast: and though both are white, yet that of virgins is thinnest, and less in quantity; neither is it so sweet. And therefore, if virgins happen to have such milk, they are not for that reason to be deemed unchaste.

Upon the whole matter, when a man marries, and finds upon lying with his wife the tokens of her virginity, he has all the reason in the world to be satisfied he has married a virgin : but if, on the contrary, he finds them not, he has no reason to suspect her of unchastity, as if she were not a virgin since the *hymen*, or *claustrium virginale*, may be broken so many other ways, and yet the woman be both virtuous and chaste.

And thus much I thought myself bound to say, in the beginning, of the female sex, who are often suspected and accused of dishonesty, when there is no reason for it.

CHAPTER II.

What a Woman ought to do, in order to Conception.

WOMEN that are desirous to have children, in order thereunto must give themselves to moderate exercise; for idleness and want of exercise are very great enemies to generation work : those that observe it, shall find that our city dames, who live high and do nothing, seldom have children, or if they have, they seldom live : whereas, the poor women, who accustom themselves to labour, have many children, and those lusty. Nor need we wonder at it, if we consider the benefit that comes by moderate exercise and labour : for it opens the pores, quickens the spirits, stirs up the natural heat, strengthens the body, senses, and comforts the limbs, and helps nature in her execrises, of which the procreation of children is not the least.

Next to moderate exercise, she must avoid all manner of discontent, and the occasion of it ; for discontent is a great enemy to conception, and contentment and quietness of mind are as great friends to it : for contentment dilates the heart and arteries, whereby the vital blood or spirit is sufficiently distributed throughout the body : and thence arise such affections as please, recreate, and refresh the nature of man, as hope, joy, love, gladness, and mirth. Nor does it only comfort and strengthen the body, but also the operations and imaginations of the mother works forcibly upon the conception of the child : and therefore women ought to take great care that their children may be well formed.

Another thing that women ought to do, in order to conception, is to keep the womb in good order; and to that end see that the menses come down as they ought to do: if they are discoloured, then they are out of order: but if the blood come down pure, then women will be very prone to conceive with child, especially if they use copulation a day or two after the monthly terms are stayed.

Another thing a woman that would conceive ought to observe is, that she use not the act of copulation too often; for satiety gluts the womb, and makes it unfit to do its office. There are two things demonstrate this: the one is, that common whores (who often use copulation) have seldom any children; the other is, that those women whose husbands have been long absent conceive very quickly after their return.

And also the time of copulation ought to be convenient, that there may be no fear or surprise; for fear hinders conception.

And then let the time of copulation be natural, and not stirred up by provocatives; and observe also, that the greater the woman's desire of copulation is, the more subject she is to conceive.

A loadstone carried about a woman causeth not only conception, but concord between man and wife.

CHAPTER III.

Things necessary for Women to observe after Conception.

WOMEN are very subject to miscarriages in the two first months after conception, because then the ligaments are weak and soon broken. To prevent which, let the woman every morning drink a good draught of sage ale, and it will do her abundance of good.

But if signs of abortion or miscarriage appear, let her lay a toast dipped in tent, in case muscadel cannot be gotten, to her navel, for this is very good: or let her take a little garden tansey, and having bruised it, sprinkle it with muscadel, and apply it to the navel, and she will find it much better. Also, tansey infused in ale, like sage ale, and a draught drank every morning, is most excellent for such women as are subject to miscarriages; also take juice of tansey, clarify it, and let the woman take a spoonful or two of it; in such cases it will be an excellent preservative against miscarriages.

Also, let the air be temperate, sleep moderate, avoid watching, and immoderate exercise, with disturbing passions, loud clamours, and filthy smells: and let her abstain from all things which may provoke either the urine or the courses, and also from all sharp and windy meats: and let a moderate diet be observed

If the excrements of the guts be retained, lenify the belly with clysters made of the decoction of mallows, violets, with sugar and common oil: or make broth of burrage, buglos, beets, mallows, and take therein a little manna. But, on the contrary, if she be troubled with a looseness of the belly, let it not be stopped without the judgment of a physician: for old uterine fluxes have a malignant quality in them, which must be evacuated and removed before the flux be stayed.

CHAPTER IV.

Of the Pleasure and Advantage of Marriage, the Impropriety of Unequal Matches, and the ruinous Effects of unlawful Love.

We have hitherto been treating of the generation of man, which is effected by man and woman in the act of coition and copulation. But this cannot be done lawfully but by those who are joined together in wedlock, according to the institution of the Creater in Paradise, when he first brought man and woman together: which being so, it necessarily leads us to treat of the pleasure and advantage of a married life.

And sure there are none who question the pleasure and advantage of a married life, but reflect on its Author, and on the time and place of its institution. The Author and Institutor of marriage was no other than the great Lord of the universe, the Creator of heaven and earth, whose wisdom was infinite, and therefore knew what was best for us, and whose goodness is equal to his wisdom, and therefore instituted marriage, as what was best for the man whom he had just created, and whom he looked upon as short of that complete happiness which he had designed him, whilst he was alone, and had not a help-mate provided for him.

The time of its institution is no less remarkable: it was whilst our first parents were clothed with that virgin purity and innocence in which they were created; it was at a time wherein they had a blessed and uninterrupted converse and communion with their great Creator, and were complete in all the perfections both of mind and body, being the lively image of Him that created them: it was at a time when they could curiously survey the several incomparable beauties and perfections of each other without sin, and knew not what it was to lust: it was at this happy time that the Almighty divided Adam from himself, and of a crooked rib made a helpmate for him; and, by instituting marriage, united him unto himself again in wedlock's sacred bands. And this must needs speak very highly in commendation of a married life.

But we have first considered only the time; now let us consider next what place it was wherein at first this marriage-knot was tied, and we shall find it was paradise: a place formed by the great Creator for delight and pleasure: and, in our usual dialect, when we would show the highest satisfaction we take, and give the greatest commendation to a place, we can ascend no higher than to affirm it was like a paradise. There are many curious delicacies and delights to please the eye and charm the ear in the gardens of princes and noblemen, but paradise did certainly out-do them all; the sacred Scriptures give this high encomium of it, "It was pleasant as the garden of God!" It was, however, in the midst of this paradise, the centre of delight and happiness, that Adam was unhappy while in a single state; and therefore marriage may very properly be styled the paradise of paradise itself.

I shall show you the love of a good wife to her husband, in an illustrious example of a queen in our own nation in former times.

King Edward the first, when he went to Palestine, for the recovery of the Holy Land, in which expedition he was very victorious and successful, took his queen along with him, who willingly accompanied him in all the dangers he exposed himself to. It so happened, that after several victories obtained by him, which made him both beloved and feared, he was wounded by a Turk with an impoisoned arrow, which all the king's physicians concluded mortal unless some human creature would suck away the impoisoned blood out of the wound; at the same time declaring, that it would be the death of the person who did it. Upon this, it was proposed to several of the courtiers; but they all waived this dangerous piece of loyalty; which, when the queen perceived that the king must die for want of such kind assistance, she, with a braveness worthy of herself, declared she was resolved to undertake the cure, and venture her own life to save the king her husband; and so accordingly sucked the poisonous matter from the wound, and thereby saved the king; and the same Divine Providence that inspired her with the generous resolution, preserved her from the apparent danger as a reward of her affection.

But that which renders marriage such a mormo, and makes it such a bugbear to our modern sparks, are those unhappy consequences that too often attend it; for there are few but see the inauspicious torches Hymen lights at every wedding, what unlucky hands link in the wedding ring, nothing but fears and jars, and discontents and jealouses: a curse as cruel, or else barrenness, are all the blessings that crown the genial bed of many. But it is not marriage that is to be blamed for this: these things are only the effects of forced and unequal matches. When greedy parents, for the sake of riches, will match a daughter that is scarcely seventeen, to an old miser that is above threescore: can any one imagine that such a conjunction can ever yield satisfaction, where the inclinations are as opposite as the months of June and January. This makes the woman (who still wants a husband, for the old miser is scarce the shadow of one) either to wish, or, may be, to contrive his death, to whom her parents thus, against her will, have yoked her: or else, to satisfy her natural inclinations, she throws herself into the arms of unlawful love: which might both have been prevented, had the greedy inconsiderate parents provided her with a suitable match. A sad instance of which truth is as follows:

There lived in Warwickshire a gentleman of very good estate, who becoming old, at the death of his first wife, thought of marrying his son and heir, then at man's estate, to the daughter of a neighbouring gentlemen, of an ancient family and good estate, who approved of the motion, and agreed to give five thousand pounds to his daughter upon her marriage with the young gontleman. No sooner had the father got a sight of the young lady but, forgetting his son, he became suitor for himself; and to obtain her, offered as much money for her, (besides settling a good jointure on her) as her father had promised to give with her to his son. This liberal offer so wrought on the lady's father, that both by persuasions and menaces he forced his daughter (who was unwilling) to marry the old gentleman. But being compelled to this unequal match, she never lived contentedly with him; for her affections wandering after other men, she gave entertainment to a young gentleman of 22 years of age, whom she liked much better than her husband, being one more suitable to her years. Then she became impatient for her husband's death, and now thought every day an age to live with him and therefore sought opportunity to cut off that thread of life which she was of opinion nature lengthened out too long; and to that end, having corrupted her maid, and the stable groom, she resolved, by their assistance, and that of her inamorato, to strangle him in his bed; which resolution (although her lover failed her, and came not at the time she appointed him, recoiling at the dismal apprehension of a fact so horrid) she executed by her servants: for watching till her husband was asleep, she let in those assassins, and then casting a long towel about his neck, she caused the groom to lie upon him that he might not struggle, whilst she and her maid, by straining the towel, stopped his breath. And now the next thing was, how to prevent the discovery of this atrocious deed; and for that purpose they carried him to another room, where a close-stool was placed, on which they set him; and when the maid and groom were both withdrawn, and the coast clear, she made such a hideous outcry in the house wringing her hands, and tearing her hair, and weeping so extremely, that none suspected her: for she alleged, that missing him some time out of bed, she went to see what was the reason he staid so long, and found him dead, sitting on his close-stool; which seeming very plausible, prevented all suspicion of his death. And being thus rid of her husband, she set a greater value upon her beauty, and quite shook off her former lover (perhaps because he had implicitly refused to be an actor in her husband's tragedy) and coming up to London made the best market of her beauty that she could. But murder is a crime that seldom goes unpunished to the grave: in two years justice overtook her, and brought to light this horrid deed of darkness. The groom (one of the actors in this fatal tragedy, being retained a servant with the son and heir of the old murdered gentleman, for whom the lady was at first designed,) with some other servants attending him to Coventry, his guilty conscience (he being in his cups) forced him upon his knees to beg forgiveness of his master, for the murder of his father, and taking him aside, acquainted him with the circumstances of it. The gentleman, though struck with horror and amazement at the discovery of so vile a fact, yet gave the groom good words, but ordered his servants to have an eye upon him, that he might not escape when he was sober, and had considered what might be the issue of the confession he made: and yet, escape he did for all their vigilance; and being got to the sea-side, was (after three attempts to put to sea, being as often forced back by the winds proving contrary) happily pursued and apprehended by his master, and brought back a prisoner to Warwick, as was soon after the lady and her gentlewoman also, who were all justly executed for that horrid murder, the lady being burnt on Wolvey-Heath, and the two servants suffering death at Warwick, leaving the world a sad example of the dismal consequences of doating love, and of unequal matches; for had this lady not been forced, through the desire of lucre in her parents, to marry the old knight, but had been married to the son, as was first intended, the old gentleman might have prevented an untimely death, and the young lady have lived with innocence and honour.

And though in many such like matches the mischief does not run so high as to break forth into adultry and murder, but the young lady, form a principle of virtue and the fear of God, curbs all her natural inclinations, and is contented with the performance of her husband (how weak soever it may be, and cold and frigid) and does preserve her chastity so pure and immaculate as not to let one wandering thought corrupt it; yet, even in this very case, the husband, conscious of the abatement of his youthful vigour, and his own weak imbecile performances of the conjugal rites, suspects his virtuous lady, and watches over her with Argus's eyes, making himself and her unhappy by his senseless jealousy; and though he happen to have children by her (which may well be, having so good ground to improve on) yet he can scarcely think they are his own: his very sleep is disturbed with dreams of cuckoldom and horns; nor dares he to keep a pack of hounds, for fear Actæon's fate should follow him. These are a few of the sad effects of old men's dotage, and unequal matches.

But let us turn the tables now and see if it be better on the other side, when a young spark of twenty-two marries a grandam of seventy years, with a wrinkled face. This, I am sure, is most unnatural. Here can be no increase, unless of gold, with oftentimes the old hag (for who can call her better, that marries a young boy to satisfy her lecherous itch, when she is just tumbling into the grave?) conveys away before marriage, to her own relations, and leaves the expectant coxcomb nothing but repentance for his portion. Pocket expences perhaps she will alow him, and for that slender wages he is bound to do the basest drudgery. But if he meet with money (which was the only motive of the match, her gold being the greatest cordial at the wedding feast he may likely squander it profusely away in rioting amongst his whores, hoping, ere long, his antiquated wife will take a voyage to another world, and leave him to his liberty: whilst old grandam, finding her money wasted, and herself despised, is filled with those resentments that jealousy, envy, and neglected love produce: wishing and hoping each day to see him in his grave, though she has almost both feet in her own. Thus, each day, they wish for each other's death, which, if it come not quickly, they often help to hasten.

But these are still excrescences of marriage, and are the errors of people marrying, and not the fault of marriage itself. For, let it be what God at first ordained, a nuptial of two hearts as well as hands, whom equal years and mutual love has first united before the parson joins their hands, and such will tell you, that mortals can enjoy no greater happiness on this side heaven.

THE MIDWIVES' VADE MECUM:

CONTAINING

PARTICULAR DIRECTIONS FOR MIDWIVES, NURSES, &c.

Those that take upon them the office of midwives ought to take care to fit themselves for that employment by the knowledge of those things that are necessary for the faithful discharge thereof. And such persons ought to be of the middle age, neither too young nor too old; and of a good habit of body, not subject to diseases, fears, or sudden frights. Nor are the qualifications assigned to a good surgeon improper for a midwife,—viz. a lady's hand, a hawk's eye, and a lion's heart; to which may be added activity of body, and a convenient strength, with caution and diligence; not subject to drowsiness or impatience. She ought also to be sober, affable, courteous, chaste, not covetous or subject to passion, but bountiful and compassionate: and, above all, she ought to be qualified as the Egyptian midwives of old, that is, to have the fear of God, which is the principal thing in every state and condition, and will furnish her on all occasions both with wisdom and discretion.

When the time of birth draws near, and the good woman finds her travailing pains begin to come upon her, let her send for her midwife in time, better too soon than too late, and get those things ready which are necessary upon such occasions. When the midwife comes, let her first find whether the true time of her labour is come; for by not properly observing this, many a child hath been spoiled, and the life of the mother endangered: or at least given double the pain needful. For unskilful midwives, not minding this, have given things to force down the child, and thereby disturbed the course of her natural labour; whereas nature works best in her own time and way. I do confess, it is somewhat difficult to know the true time of some women's labour, they being troubled with pains long before their true labour comes, even some weeks before; the reason of which I conceive to be the heat of their reins; and this may be readily known by the swelling of their legs; and therefore, when women with child find their legs swell much, they may be assured that their reins are too hot. For the cure whereof, let them cool the reins before the time of their labour with oil of poppies, and oil of violets, or water lilies, by anointing the reins of their backs with them; for such women whose reins are over hot have usually hard labours. But in this case, above all the remedies that I know, I prefer the decoction of them in water; and then, having strained and clarified it with the white of an egg, boil it into a syrup with its equal weight of sugar, and keep it for use.

There are two skins that compass the child in the womb, the one is the *amnios*, and this is the inner skin; the other is the *allantois*, and this the skin that holds the urine of the child during the time that it abides in the womb. Both these skins, by the violent stirring of the child near the time of the birth, are broken; and then the urine and sweat of the child contained in them fall down to the neck of the womb; and this is that which the midwives call *the waters*, and is an infallible sign that the birth is very near; for the child is no more able to subsist in the womb after those skins are broken, than a naked man is in the cold air. These waters, if the child come presently after them, facilitate the labour, by making the passage slippery; and therefore the midwife must have a care that she force not the waters away, for nature knows better the true time of the birth than she, and usually retains the waters till that time.

SOME GENUINE RECIPES

FOR

CAUSING SPEEDY DELIVERY.

A LOADSTONE held in the labouring woman's hand. Take wild tansey, bruise and apply it to the woman's nostrils. Take also date stones and beat them to powder, and let her take half a dram of them in white wine at a time.

Take parsley, bruise it, and press out the juice, and put it up (being so dipped) into the mouth of the womb, and it will presently causes the child to come away, though it be dead, and the after burden also; besides, it cleanseth the womb, and also the child in the womb, of all gross humours.

Let no midwife ever force away a child, unless she is sure it is dead. I once was where a woman was in labour, which being very hard, her midwife sent for another midwife to assist her, which midwife sending the first down stairs, and designing to have the honour of delivering the woman herself, forced away the body of the child, and left the head behind: of which the woman was forced afterwards to be delivered by a man midwife.

After the child is born, great care is to be taken by the midwife in cutting the navel string, which, though by some is accounted but a trifle, yet it requires none of the least skill of a midwife, to do it with that prudence and judgment that is requisite. And that it may be done so, you must consider, as soon as the child is freed from its mother, whether it be weak or strong; but if the child be weak, put back gently part of the vital and natural blood in the body of the child by its navel (for both the vital and natural spirits are communicated by the mother to the child by its navel string;) for that doth much recruit a weak child; but if the child be strong you may forbear.

As to the manner of cutting the child's navel-string, let the ligature or binding be very strong; and be sure not to cut it off very near the binding, lest the binding unloose. You need not fear to bind the navel-string very hard, because it is void of sense, and that part of the navel-string which you leave on falls of its own accord in a few days; the whole course of nature being now changed in the child, it having another way ordained to nourish it. It is no matter with what instrument you cut it off, if it be sharp and you do it cleverly. The piece of the navel-string that falls off, be sure you keep it from touching the ground; remember what I have before told you concerning this matter, and if you keep it by you it may be of use. The navel-string being thus cut off, put a little cotten or lint to the place, to keep it warm, lest the cold enter the body of the child, which it will be apt to do if it be not bound up hard enough.

The next thing to be done, is to bring away the after birth, or secundine, else it will be very dangerous for the woman.— But this must be done by gentle means, and without delay, for in this case especially delays are dangerous; and whatever I have set down before, as good to cause speedy delivery, and bring away the birth, is good also to bring away the afterbirth.

And after the birth and after-birth, are brought away, if the woman's body be weak, keep her not too warm; for extremity of heat doth weaken nature, and dissolves the strength; but whether she be weak or strong, let no cold air come nearer her at first; for cold is an enemy to the spermatic parts. If cold gets into the womb, it increases the after-pains, causes swellings in the womb, and does great hurt to the nerves.

If what I have written be carefully observed by midwives, and such nurses as keep women in their lying-in, by God's blessing the child-bed women may do very well, and both midwife and nurse gain credit and reputation. For though these directions may in some things thwart the common practice, yet they are grounded upon experience, and will infallibly answer the end.

But there are several accidents that lying-in women are subject unto, which must be provided against; and these I shall speak of next.

The first I shall mention are after-pains, about the cause of which, authors very much differ: some think they are caused by the thinness, some by the thickness, some by the slimness, and others by the sharpness of the blood: but my own opinion is, they proceed from cold and water. But whatever the cause may be, this I know, that if my foregoing directions be observed, they will be very much abated, if not quite taken away. But in case they do happen, boil an egg, and pour out the yolk of it, with which mix a spoonful of cinnamon-water, and let her drink of it ; and if you mix it with two grains of ambergris, it will be better.

The second accident lying-in women are subject to is excoriation in the lower part of the womb. To help this, use oil of sweet almonds, or rather oil of St. John's wort, to anoint the part with.

Another accident is, that sometimes, through very hard labour, and great straining to bring the child into the world, the lying-in woman comes to be troubled with the hemorrhoids or piles To cure this, let her use polypodium bruised and boiled in her meat and drink.

A fourth thing that often follows is, the retention of the menses; this is very dangerous, and if not remedied proves mortal But for this, let her take such medicines as strongly provoke the terms: and such are peony roots, dittany, juniper berries, centuary sage savory, pennyroyal, feverfew.

The last thing I shall mention is, the overflowing of the menses. This happens not so often as the foregoing, but yet sometimes it does ; and in such cases take shepherd's purse, either boiled in any convenient liquor, or dried and beaten to powder, and you will find it very good to stop them.

Having thus finished my Vade-Mecum for midwives, before I conclude I will add something of the choice and qualifications of a good nurse: that those who have occasion for them, may know how to order themselves, for the good of the children whom they nurse.

First, then, if you would choose a good nurse, choose one of a sanguine complexion, not only because that complexion is generally the best, but also because all children in their minority have their complexion predominent. And that you may know such a woman, take the following description of her.

Her stature of the middle size, her body fleshy, but not fat ; but of a merry, pleasant, and cheerful countenance · a fresh ruddy colour, and her skin so very clear that you may see her veins through it. She is one that loves company, and never cares to be alone · never given to anger, but much inclined to playing and singing : and, which makes her the fittest person for a nurse, she very much delights in children. In choosing such a one, you can hardly do amiss· only let me give you this caution, if you cannot get one exactly of this description [which you will find very difficult] get one as near to it as you can. And let these rules further guide you in your choice.

1. Let her age be between 20 and 30, for then she is in her prime.

2. Let her be in health, for her sickness infects her milk, and her milk the child.

3. Let her be a prudent women, for such a one will be careful of her child.

4. Let her not be too poor; for if she wants, the child must want too.

5. Let her be well bred; for ill bred nurses corrupt good nature.

6. If it be a boy that is to be nursed, let the nurse be such a one whose last child was a boy, and so it will be more agreeable; but if it be a girl, let the nurse be one whose last child was a girl.

7. If the nurse has a husband, see that he be a good likely man, and not given to debauchery; for that may have an influence upon the child.

8. In the last place, let the nurse take care she be not with child herself: for if so, she must of necessity either spoil her own, or yours, or both.

To a nurse thus qualified, you may put your child without danger. And let such a nurse take the following directions, for the better governing and ordering herself in that station.

Approved Directions for Nurses.

1. LET her use her body to exercise. If she hath nothing else to do, let her exercise hersslf by dancing the child; for moderate exercise causeth good digestion; and I am sure good blood must needs make good milk, and good milk cannot fail of making a thriving child.

2. Let her live in good air; there is nothing more material than this. It is the want of this makes so many children die in London; and even those few that live are not of the best constitutions, for gross and thick air makes unwieldy bodies and dull wits: And let none wonder at this; for the operation of the air, to the body of man, is as great as meat and drink, for it helps to engender the vital and animal spirits; and is thus the cause of sickness and of health, of life and death.

3. Let her be careful of her diet, and avoid all salt meats, garlics, leeks, onions, and mustard, excessive drinking of wine, strong beer, or ale, for they trouble the child's body with choler: cheese, both new and old, afflicts it with melancholy, and all fish with phlegm.

4. Let her never deny herself sleep when she is drowsy, for by that means she will be more wakeful when the child cries.

5. Let her avoid all disquiets of mind, anger, vexation, sorrow, and grief; for these things very much disorder a woman, and therefore must needs be hurtful to the milk.

6. If the nurse's milk happen to be corrupted by an accident, as sometimes it may be, being either too hot or too cold, in such cases let her diet be good, and let her observe the cautions which have already been given her. And then, if her milk be too hot, let her cool it with endive, succory, lettuce, sorrel, purslain, and plantain; if it be too cold, let her use beverage, vervain, buglos, mother of thyme, and cinnamon; and let her observe this general rule, that whatsoever strengthens the child in the womb, the same attends the milk.

7. If the nurse wants milk, the thistle, commonly called our lady's thistle, is an excellent thing, for her breeding of milk, there being few things growing (if any) that breed more and better milk than that doth; also the hoofs of the forefeet of the cow, dried and beaten to powder, and a dram of the powder taken every morning in any convenient liquor, increases milk.

Choice Remedies for increasing Milk.

If a nurse be given to much fretting, it makes her lean, and hinders digestion. and she can never have store of milk, nor what she hath be good. Bad meats and drinks also hinder the increase of milk, and therefore ought to be forborne. A woman that would increase her milk, should eat the best of food (that is, if she can get it,) and let her drink milk wherein fennel seed have been steeped. Let her drink barley water, and burrage, and spinach; also goat's milk, cow's milk, and lamb sodden with verjuice. Let her also comfort the stomach with confection of anniseed, caraway and cummin seeds, also use those seeds sodden in water; also take barley water, and boil therein green fennel and dill, and sweeten it with sugar, and drink it at pleasure.

Hot fomentations open the breasts, and attract the blood, as the decoction of fennel, smallage, or stamped mint applied, Or,

Take fennel and parsley, green, each a handful, boil and stamp them, and barley meal half an ounce, gith seed a dram, storax, calamint, two drams oil of lilies two ounces, and make a poultice.

Lastly, Take half an ounce of deer's suet, and as much parsley roots, an ounce and a half of barley meal, three drams of red storax, and three ounces of oil of sweet almonds; boil the roots well, and beat them to pap, then mingle the other amongst them, and put it warm to the nipples, and it will increase the milk.

And thus courteous reader, I have at length finished what I designed, and what I promised; and can truly affirm, that thou hast here those recipes, remedies, and directions given unto thee, with respect to childbearing women, midwives, and nurses, that are worth their weight in gold, and will assuredly (with the blessing of God) answer the end, whensoever thou hast occasion to make use of them, they not being things taken on trust from tradition or hearsay, but the result and dictates of sound reason and long experience.

END OF THE LAST LEGACY.

CONCLUSION.

Courteous Reader,

In the Works of the renowned and famous philosopher, Aristotle, you have got laid before you a Collection of the best Observations on the Secrets of Nature, that ever the World was favoured with on that subject. Let me now entreat you, who have read them, and all those who may hereafter do so, to mark well what is therein contained, and thereby direct your future conduct, which you will find to your advantage. Whatever young and inconsiderate persons may think or say of what is herein contained, it is absolutely necessary to be known; and, when reduced to practice, may prove the happy means of preventing many fatal and lamentable consequences, which ignorance and inconsideration produce. Farewell.

THE END.

www.ingramcontent.com/pod-product-compliance
Ingram Content Group UK Ltd.
Pitfield, Milton Keynes, MK11 3LW, UK
UKHW022028300325
456881UK00006B/69